The Insp

Finding Joy While
Caring for Those You Love

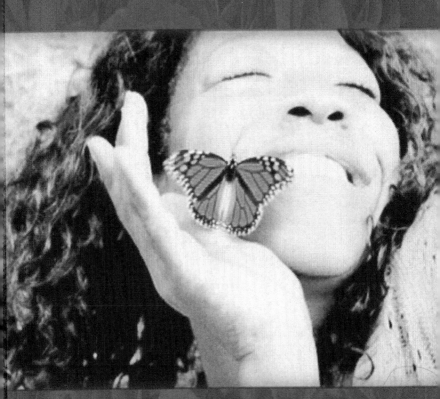

Peggi Speers • Tia Walker

The Inspired Caregiver – Finding Joy While Caring for Those You Love

www.TheInspiredCaregiver.com

Flowspirations LLC.
395 Del Monte Center, Ste 182
Monterey, CA 93940

Cover Photo: Ruth Wishengrad
Cover Model: Tia Walker
Cover Design: Sheila Shaw
Photograph of Tia and Peggi and of Peggi: Hugh Browne
Peggi's Hair Stylist: Sandra Haven at SC Studios
Photograph of Tia in Bio: Edward Clynes

ISBN: 148232959X
ISBN: 9781482329599
Library of Congress Control Number: 2013902229
CreateSpace Independent Publishing Platform
North Charleston, South Carolina

First Edition

*To the Unsung Heroes
of the World:
Caregivers*

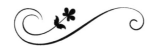

Contents

Journey of a Caregiver – Peggi's Story

"Where there is ruin, there is hope for a treasure."

~Rumi

"It's either Rose or me," I reasoned as I quickly backed into my driveway and popped the hatchback open while my dear friend Sheila lifted Rose's suitcase and slipped it into my car, quietly closing the hatchback.

Rose tried to see the action she heard behind her, but the seatbelt locked her closely to her seat. "Where are we? What are we doing?" she sharply asked.

I slammed my foot down on the gas pedal, and we darted away as I distracted Rose by replying, "We're going to get a decaf cappuccino at Starbucks."

This confused her even more. In actuality, now that I had her clothes, medication, and toiletries, I planned to drive her down the coast until the new medication kicked in and she was sedated enough for me to take to the assisted living facility. This would be my second try. The first attempt had been unsuccessful. She had stormed around the facility like a soldier, cursing me and shouting that she was not going to stay there. The owner then told me, "She cannot stay here tonight. She needs different medication to sedate her. She is a fighter."

Never in my wildest dreams would I have imagined breaking the law of my soul by lying to and deceiving Rose, my dear friend and second mother. Here I was, sneaking sedatives into her breakfast as though I was a secret agent from an episode of *Mission: Impossible* and answering her repeated and endless questions with imaginative, believable lies in a desperate attempt to save my own life. With or without her approval, she was moving out of my home and into the assisted living villa that I had painstakingly found for her after researching every other option available.

I met Rose and her husband Dieter almost thirty years ago while vacationing in Hawaii with my mother. I was only thirteen then, and we immediately connected with this very positive couple. As fate would have it, they lived only a few hours from us, and by spending a day together once every other month, we were able to continue our friendship. Rose and Dieter had both survived World War II in Germany. They rarely discussed their past. They had only one other set of friends, a Brazilian couple Rose later "wrote off." Due to their hidden scars, Rose and Dieter didn't trust anyone, so we considered our friendship a privilege. Dieter always had a smile on his face and loved to remind us, "These are the good ol' days." We spent our time together living in the now, enjoying good food, a beautiful view, and each other. It was a simple, accepting friendship of love and laughter, and we cherished every moment.

After Dieter and my mother passed away, Rose was dependent on me for support and friendship. It was a given that if anything happened to Rose, I would be the one to care for her and her two cats. Looking back, I wonder what my life would have been like if I had not raced from Monterey to San Francisco to check on Rose's well-being. She wasn't answering her phone, though she knew I would be calling her at nine p.m. after I returned from my weekend conference. She never missed my call. What if I had waited until morning and found her lying on the floor after four nights and four days, instead of three nights and four days? Would she have survived? Rose and I may have been spared the disturbing joke life played—having us spend endless hours, days, and energy working together with her medical teams to accomplish what many whispered could not be done: Rose learning to walk and use her arm again, as if she had never experienced both a stroke and heart attack. With sheer determination, we accomplished that, only to have her mind slip into the disease of dementia.

Had I waited until morning to find her, I may have been spared the hurtful words she frequently barked. "You are not a queen." "You are not your mother! You will never be your mother!" "I wish you were in my place!" "I run you over!" "You are not the girl I met years ago!" I wouldn't have had to endure hearing her disown me several times a day, shouting, "I write you off!" Then, after realizing she couldn't remember who her friends were or where she was, she would revoke that statement and laugh, "Oh, I can't write you off. I have no one else."

I may not have had to experience this caregiver horror movie with Rose trying to walk out of my home, accusing me of trying to keep her locked up. She forgot that almost every day we went out for a wonderful lunch, drove the coastline to give her a sense of freedom, and went to physical therapy appointments where the therapists doted on her. I may not have had to endure the many unprovoked silent treatments or glares so potent they sent me dashing to my bedroom, curling up in my bed, waiting for the nausea to pass.

If I had only waited until morning, perhaps Rose would have been spared the misery of feeling confused, insulted, and powerless. Perhaps she would not have experienced her greatest fear—losing her memory and being locked up in an assisted living facility or nursing home. Perhaps she would have gone to a place of eternal peace instead of struggling with a new life she hated. Every single morning, Rose said (purposely loud enough for me to hear), "Is this my life? I hate my life. I kill myself."

Dementia is a cruel disease for everyone involved, especially the caregiver. With some of us, it's almost as though our loved ones vacate their bodies several times a day, and dark spirits move in to misbehave physically and verbally, causing us so many sleepless nights, pain, and anguish.

Though I have been an Inspired Caregiver for loved ones suffering from cancer and renal failure, I was untrained and unprepared for the caregiving journey I would walk with Rose. Had it not been for my faith, friends, family, Rose's medical team, wellness coaches, and advice from those working in assisted living facilities, I am not confident I would be here today.

I do know one thing. If I had waited until morning to check on Rose, and she had not survived, this book never would have been written. I wouldn't have experienced such great love, great laughter, great hope, great hopelessness, great despair, and great awakenings. I would not have discovered the secret of being an inspired anything in life and I would not have met the many incredible people who contributed so much to my caregiving adventure and this book. I definitely would not have witnessed the inspiring power of sheer determination as Rose chanted, "Ich kann! Ich will! Ich muss!" (I can! I will! I must!) at every challenge she faced.

These pages were co-created with my dear friend Tia, who also walked the caregiving path with both her parents and with me emotionally. Unbeknownst to Tia, at times she carried me through some challenging moments just by listening when I needed to express my feelings of shock and injustice, giving me objective feedback and support. Never underestimate the power of listening and sincere, loving support and encouragement. It can change our world.

It is our hope that you find the courage and willpower to practice the art of self-care on a consistent basis. May you find comfort, encouragement, guidance, and inspiration throughout these pages. And most of all, may you feel joy every single day!

~Peggi

Journey of a Caregiver – Tia's Story

"One person caring about another represents life's greatest value."

~Jim Rohn

My journey to the place of "caregiver" was quite unexpected, and something I never thought I'd experience in my twenties. Little did I know what profound effect of having both my parents face health challenges would have on my life. In hindsight, it was one of my biggest gifts and a time of great personal growth. Yet at the time, I felt fear, sadness, and a sense of helplessness.

My father was a "self-made" man, a healthy entrepreneur. To see him vulnerable was difficult. The daughter he once provided for now provided for him. This was a life-changing experience for both of us. I saw a side of him I had never seen. It takes tremendous courage to surrender, soften, and allow another to care for you. I now have so much compassion for those taking care of their loved ones. I admire the very noble caregiving professionals who care for those they are not related to.

I remember my mother as vibrant, loving, tenacious, creative, and deeply in love with her family. She was someone I admired, who was always in my corner—someone I could count on. It was heart wrenching to see such vibrancy dulled by multiple medical conditions and the sheer exhaustion from her determination to keep it together "just one more day." Good days were the fuel that kept me smiling when the bad days occurred. My mother referred to herself humorously as a "Friday car." These are the cars built at the end of a long week, perhaps with a little less attention paid to the assembly. I appreciated her sense of humor, which I continue to draw on when life hands me lemons.

Her encounter with the medical system provided me much insight and confirmed the importance of taking your health into your own hands. I became frustrated dealing with a system that, at times, made no sense whatsoever. This propelled me to seek out alternatives to western medicine. When I was faced with my own medical challenges, I found a homeopathic physician who used less invasive treatments with fewer side effects.

Imagine owning a classic Ferrari and ignoring regular maintenance, fueling up with cheap gas, and allowing anyone who says they know the way to your destination to drive it. This seems ridiculous, yet we are gifted these price-less machines, these amazing assemblies of complex systems, our bodies, which we sometimes ignore and turn the care of over to others. Where in your lives are you working to the point of imbalance and stress? Where do you ingest medications without fully knowing the side effects? How easy is it for you to turn over decisions about your health care when you are depleted and overwhelmed? I learned from my mom's experience and said, "No more," and then took control and responsibility for my own health.

The Inspired Caregiver is designed to inspire caregiving in a new way. Instead of caring from a place of obligation, care from a place of love: love for the ones we care for and love for ourselves. I believe one's highest achievement is ser-vice—service to others while honoring and loving oneself.

I have always felt that whatever challenges we face, when we look through lenses of compassion and love for ourselves and others, challenges can become inspira-tions. When asked to co-create *The Inspired Caregiver*, which was the heart's calling of my dear friend Peggi, I knew the importance of the tips, information, and re-sources we would provide to others who, like me, were faced with the sometimes overwhelming challenge of caring for another. It is from that space of sharing and a "we're all in this together" perspective that we share our real world, real solutions with you. I hope you find inspiration throughout and you take that inspiration to be inspired in all areas of your life. You can do it!

~Tia

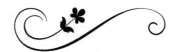

I Didn't Sign Up For This!

*"There are only four kinds of people in this world—
those who have been caregivers, those who currently
are caregivers, those who will be caregivers, and those
who will need caregivers."*

~Rosalynn Carter

What do you do when a role you didn't sign up for chooses you? Sometimes being a caregiver happens overnight, changing and redefining our lives. We are faced with little training and a great weight on our shoulders. Perhaps our child is born with special needs or demands. Perhaps our parents have developed Alzheimer's or another form of dementia, or our spouses have had accidents and can no longer walk. Whatever the case, it is our love for them and their well-being that has assigned us to the extremely honorable, yet taxing position of caregiver.

How we respond to these responsibilities will ultimately determine our physical, emotional, mental, spiritual, and financial health, as well as the health of the persons for whom we are caring. It is not uncommon for caregivers to experience financial devastation, develop an illness, feel isolated, and even become emotionally bankrupt, all signs of caregiver burnout, or "overwhelm." Overwhelm can lead to patient abuse, so it is important not only to strive to become an excellent caregiver, but to be an inspired one, as well!

While writing this book, we discovered that it holds THE secret to becoming an Inspired Caregiver, parent, teacher, writer, speaker, student, psychologist, lawyer, politician, medical doctor, minister, scientist, spouse, CEO, or any other role or profession. *To be an inspired anything, we must consistently live in our centers by practicing the art of self-care every single day. By doing so, it is easier to care for our loved ones, clients, and customers from a place of love, compassion, and patience.*

Becoming an Inspired Caregiver may not be easy, but it is achievable. As you are inspired in all that you do, you live a life that is full of joy and purpose, regardless of the situation. We encourage you to train your body and mind with the same dedication a professional athlete takes when training for a long-distance marathon, because you might be! You may provide care for a short time or for many years. You may sacrifice time and money, and use most of your energy to keep up with seemingly impossible demands. If we were patients needing caregivers, we would want our caregivers to be inspired ones—giving us the best care possible while taking care of their own health, as well.

Inspired Caregivers understand and accept that our responsibilities have changed drastically and we must make our well-being a priority, as we have never done before. Our goal is to support you in all stages of your caregiving journey. We especially encourage those of you suffering from overwhelm to become like the phoenix, rising from the emotional ashes after being burnt out from demands and responsibilities that have been placed upon you for far too long.

It is our hope that you become your own source of inspiration while serving your loved ones. The tips in this book, if implemented, will not only help you to become the best caregiver you can be, they just might save YOUR life.

How to Use This Book:

Throughout these pages, you will find questions, which are our invitation for you to be in inquiry and to spark thoughts you haven't had. Taking the time to answer these questions on the lines provided will help you become an Inspired Caregiver. You will be reminded that self-care is a priority and **THE** path to sustaining yourself when you are called to care beyond your expectations.

The quotes are wonderful reminders and another source of inspiration. You might find a quote that provides the words you need to lift your spirit and help you achieve all that you feel called to do. Affirmations are your mental vitamins, providing supplementary positive thoughts that you need to balance the barrage of negative events and thoughts you experience daily. Incorporating affirmations in your daily practice is a great way to show self-care.

Use this book to guide you to live continuously in your center. Allow it to give you permission to make self-care your priority. Carry it with you to doctors' appointments to read when you need understanding and support. Allow it to remind you that you are not alone on this caregiving pilgrimage and that there is support for you every step of the way.

Important:

You may notice a common theme of self-care. This is done purposely to make your subconscious mind aware of the danger of allowing yourself to slip out-of-balance and into the infection of caregiver overwhelm.

Please Note:

Though this book references different faiths, we do not promote any specific religion. You are invited to take your guidance from wherever you draw your inspiration.

Are You a Caregiver?

"I believe that most caregivers find that they inherit a situation where they just kind of move into caregiving. It's not a conscious decision for most caregivers, and they are ultimately left with the responsibility of working while still trying to be the caregiver, the provider, and the nurturer."

~Sharon, caregiver of twenty years

"Caregiver: a person who cares for a child or for someone who is sick or disabled"
Random House *Webster's Dictionary*

<u>Identify Your Role: Are you a Caregiver?</u> If you are helping someone with a health challenge, you are a caregiver. You are giving care.

For over twenty years, Sharon didn't realize she was a caregiver. Although she was consumed with her husband's illness and was the "provider, nurse, financial person, and nurturer of the family," it wasn't until years later, after feeling frustrated, depressed, and resentful, that she had an awakening and realized she was "too young to die alive."

"I didn't even identify my role as a caregiver. It's only been in the last six months, looking back at my life, that I've accepted and realized I've spent many years as a caregiver. My illusion or disillusion of a caregiver was someone who was taking care of another who was bedridden. This is not true. The average caregiver is a woman who's working full time and taking care of someone else 20% of the time."

Sharon's story is, unfortunately, common. In the United States, nearly one out of every four households has an unpaid family caregiver of someone over the age of fifty. When we take care of those we love, we sometimes minimize the responsibility. The overriding thought, "This is what I'm supposed to do: help my family when they need me," doesn't honor or prepare us for the enormous job we've actually taken. Often we have no training and accept the job out of obligation or love for someone needing care. The first step to becoming an Inspired Caregiver is to recognize that you are a caregiver.

What are the ways you can be considered a caregiver?

_____

_____

_____

_____

_____

_____

*I am a caregiver and I lovingly care for others
while honoring myself.*

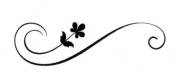

Accepting Your Role as a Caregiver

"Our suffering is directly related to our resistance to what is. When you resist what is, you suffer. When you accept what is, you do what you have to do."

~Cheryl Richardson *www.CherylRichardson.com*

It is extremely important that once we recognize we are caregivers, we must either accept it or relinquish the role to someone else. What is "accepting it?" It is acknowledging that we are responsible for another's care and they depend on us. It is also letting go of any resistance to doing what we have been called to do. Caregiving is part of the cycle of life, and once we accept this role and are willing to do whatever we can to help, we must accept that, for a while at least, our lives and priorities have a new focus, a new mission that dominates every day.

Once we have accepted our roles as caregivers on the deepest level of our souls, we must develop spirits of sacrifice and service. By replacing our personal goals and ambitions with our well-being as our first priorities, and the care of our loved ones as the second priorities, many other aspirations are held in a delicate balance. Sometimes those goals and aspirations are on hold indefinitely. In most cases, if we continue to make personal goals our priorities, we can create an enormous amount of unnecessary stress for ourselves physically, mentally, and emotionally. Pursuing projects and goals that require more of us than we have to give is a recipe for disaster, which often results in developing overwhelm.

Understand that we must view this responsibility as a professional athlete would, claiming our proper rest, feeding our bodies the nutrients we need to endure the seemingly never-ending demands, and taking, at the very least, twenty minutes three times a week to exercise. Because we are running marathons, perhaps for the long haul, this is non-negotiable. Allowing ourselves to be unbalanced mentally, physically, and emotionally may result in the loss of our lives.

~ *REAL WORLD EXAMPLE OF ACCEPTING NEW PRIORITIES* ~

Sarah was attending college full time and working when her mother was struck by a car. Due to the accident, her mother now needed a high level of care. Sarah's father had previously passed away, and she was an only child. Sarah knew the enormity of what she was about to take on. To stay in balance, Sarah postponed her studies to concentrate on her own health, her mother's healing, and her job, which was one of her main sources of income. When her mother began to heal and became more self-sufficient, Sarah was able to slowly add classes to her schedule and eventually attend college full time again. Sarah's ability to prioritize her life allowed her to transition into her role as a caregiver with grace and ease.

Have you truly accepted your role as a caregiver? How can you arrange your priorities to help you move forward in the spirit of love and confidence?

_____

_____

_____

_____

_____

_____

I have the opportunity to serve as a caregiver.
I am accepting of all that is.

The Inspired Caregiver Pledge

I know I have what it takes to become an Inspired Caregiver! I now dedicate myself to consistently care for my physical, mental, spiritual, and emotional health on a daily basis. I understand that I am my loved one's advocate, and to give _____ my very best, I must be at my best.

I train my mind and body as an athlete would, feeding it with the proper nutrients, water, rest, and exercise for endurance and strength. I am courageous. Therefore, I participate in counseling and caregiver support groups on a regular basis to obtain the emotional stability I need to live a healthy, joyful life, despite the pressures around me. I give myself permission to take the time I need every week to participate in activities that rejuvenate, replenish, and renew my mind, body, and soul.

I understand that the past is over and there's no turning back! I accept my new responsibilities and goals with enthusiasm and inspiration. I am focused. I am determined. I am successful. Yes! And so it is.

Set Up Your Foundation ASAP

"The first defense against drama is a schedule, a regular routine."

~Julia Cameron

Heed the 5 Ps: Proper Planning Promotes Peak Performance

In the beginning, while you have the energy to move mountains, set up your foundation. Most of us start out as Inspired Caregivers. We want to help! We are needed! Our loved ones depend on us for their well-being; perhaps we are their heroes and their only hope. We are solution oriented, smart, capable people! We can help! We will help! We will not let them down! The time to become organized and informed is when we are in this power of accelerated energy. We owe it to ourselves to take action and set up our foundations immediately, taking this responsibility as seriously as if we were running successful businesses.

In business, many failures are not due to employee incompetence, but to the systems, they are required to follow. And so it is with the business of caregiving. If we set up an effective system where another family member and/or friend can take our place, they, too, will be able to give proper care to our loved ones in our absence. We believe this is one of the main secrets to caregiving success.

Below are some tips essential to your caregiving foundation:

1. **Create an Inspired Caregiver Team Binder** in which everything is documented throughout the day. This is especially helpful if you have siblings helping with the care.

The Essential Resource –
An Inspired Caregiver Team Binder

~PEGGI'S STORY~

When my mother was bedridden, my sisters and I cared for her in shifts around the clock. My sister Anne (RN, CCRN) started a communication binder, which we now call the Inspired Caregiver Team Binder. It was mandatory that we consult this binder before we began our shift. Not only did it contain all of the contact numbers we needed, including personal cell phone numbers, it also provided notes from the previous shift and a place for us to write pertinent information, such as when her medications were taken and what medications were given to her. We were required to write down any other information, such as how she was feeling mentally or physically, and any concerns or comments. This binder became a sacred tool, as it kept us all on "the same page" (no pun intended) when it came to our mother's medical condition.

I used a binder when I cared for Rose, as well, which was a lifesaver (perhaps literally). Her doctor would ask me questions requiring such detailed answers; I would have to go back and refer to the information I documented in the binder in order to answer her accurately.

2. **Become proactive with your loved one's medical team and social worker.** The social worker can help you with medical insurance information, direct you to resources you may need, and refer you to organizations and individuals who can help. Have a section in your Inspired Caregiver Team Binder devoted to the information they give you. Know the answers to questions like: What does Medicare cover? What does Medicaid cover? What coverage is available to you? What organizations can help? Where can you apply for grants?

3. **Create an Inspired Caregiver Team** that consists of your loved one's medical team, social worker, wellness coach, caregiving support group, assisted living manager and their caregivers, and anyone essential to helping with your loved one's care and your health during your caregiving journey. Place their information and notes in your Inspired Caregiver Team Binder.

4. **Make sure your loved ones have a medical alert card and/or bracelet on them at all times.** In an emergency, our minds can freeze, and with a bracelet or medical alert card, we don't have to remember what medications our loved ones have taken or the contact numbers of their medical teams. If we are not with them and they cannot speak for themselves in an emergency, the

card or bracelet will inform help of their medical needs and provide our contact information. For a free Medical Alert Card download, visit www. TheInspiredCaregiver.com

5. **Become an expert on the condition of your loved one**. Ask your loved one's medical team what you can expect if his or her condition declines, and what tools, equipment, or resources you will need. We are not advocating you expect the worst, but it is helpful to be prepared with the knowledge you need, should your loved one's health take an unpleasant turn, especially if your loved one suffers from dementia.

Many of us who care for a loved one suffering from dementia have no idea what to expect from this disease. Instead of living in our loved ones' world and just going along with it, we drain our energy by constantly reminding our care recipients of the reality of the situation, frustrating and confusing them and, therefore, risking verbal abuse. If our loved ones believe they are on a cruise ship or in the year 1901, by just going along with it, we may escape their abuse and actually have fun.

6. **Find organizations in your area that can help with your specific needs.** If we work and our loved ones will be home alone, a resource similar to the Amherst H. Wilder Foundation (www. wilder.org) can be invaluable. Organizations like

this can help find transportation as well as offer personal coaching. We strongly encourage using the coaching services from your local caregiver resource center. There are organizations that offer daily classes for loved ones recovering from strokes, as well as sitters who can stay and entertain our loved ones while you are gone. Foundations that offer classes and lunches to individuals over the age of sixty from nine a.m. to five p.m., Monday through Friday, are also available. Browse the Internet for local resources and ask your loved one's medical team if the medical center offers programs that address your needs.

7. **Become an expert with any equipment your loved one needs**, such as the wheelchair. If at the peak of a stressful moment, your loved one's wheelchair breaks or does something that prevents you from pushing it, you will know how to troubleshoot it immediately. An excellent time-saving source is youtube.com. There you may find easy-to-comprehend, step-by-step instructional videos on the exact equipment you have.

8. **Seek software and electronics that may help you and/or your loved one.** We once received an email from a caregiver who purchased the Presto Mail Service for her mother. This service provides a place family and friends can send emails,

photographs, and e-cards to their loved ones. No computer required! There is nothing new for the loved one to learn; messages and photographs are automatically received and printed. It is a great tool for those who do not use a computer, and it has made her mother very happy, and therefore, easier to care for.

9. **Look into the FMLA**. If you are employed and caring for an immediate family member (spouse, child, or parent) with a serious health condition, you may want to look into the Family and Medical Leave Act (FMLA), which provides certain employees with up to twelve weeks of unpaid, job-protected leave per year. It also requires that your group health benefits be maintained during the leave.

   Barbara lived in California and had to travel to Maine to care for her mother, who suffered from cancer. She was able to take time off without jeopardizing her job and kept her benefits during this very difficult time.

10. **Consider banking on-line.** Banking on-line is an excellent time saver. Bills can be automatically paid, reducing run-around time. A banker can coach you through the process, if needed.*

11. <u>**Recruit at least one friend and/or family member to help you obtain all the information, resources, equipment, and tools you'll need to assemble this list!**</u> Have your recruit or recruits help you get organized! Create a plan together, including a system for house cleaning, cooking, medication management, and other matters while they too are energized and motivated.

~*TIPS FOR THE ORGANIZATION-CHALLENGED CAREGIVER*~

Not an organizer? You are not alone. Sometimes creative minds, or just feeling overwhelmed, can paralyze us. When paralysis sets in, we don't do the things we know we should do. Success is sometimes as simple as taking a tiny first step.

Writing one or two little tasks a day on your calendar and doing them helps you build your foundation. Use this book as your reference and check off the things you have completed. Some days you may only have the energy to buy the binder or call a friend or family member and ask if he or she will be a part of your Inspired Caregiving Team by relieving you for an hour or two when necessary.

Hire a professional organizer or a personal assistant for a couple hours to jumpstart what needs to be done. These individuals can be found in local directories. Spending a small amount to help maintain your health by reducing your stress is worth it. If you are short on cash, think outside the box; ask for volunteers from your church and/or place an ad on Craigslist to sell something that no longer serves you.

We recommend reading Time Warrior, by Steve Chandler. This is an excellent book for the organization-challenged caregiver and those needing help with time management. One of Steve's suggestions is: "Dissolve worry and anxiety by taking action. What's my next action? And then, doing that action now. Action. Movement. Decisive energy. Solves most everything."

It is important to be assertive when laying our foundations to efficient caregiving. If we procrastinate and do not organize little things in the beginning, they will become mountains later, spiraling us into overwhelm. This happens when we allow ourselves to become off-center, which, like alcoholism and obesity, may sneak up on us almost overnight. In overwhelm, where before we were solution-oriented individuals, we may now feel overwhelmed and hopeless. Once filled with energy, we may feel sick or exhausted. Once filled with inspiration, joy, and gentleness, we may feel irritated, impatient, and even abusive. By immediately taking the action needed to create a strong foundation, we will live healthier, solution-oriented, and energetic lives while giving our best to our loved ones and ourselves. This is what being an Inspired Caregiver is all about.

Have you created your Inspired Caregiver Team and built your foundation? If not, who can you recruit to help you right away?

_____

_____

_____

_____

_____

_____

I have built a strong foundation. The good work I did early on has made my job as a caregiver easier. My caregiver team supports me.

* Please see our reference page regarding banking on-line.

Ask and It Is Given

Facebook – An Inspired Caregiver's Communication Tool

"What you are seeking is seeking you."

~Rumi

It is said that it takes a village to raise a child, and we would like to add that it takes a village to help us walk the path of caregiving, as well. Our village includes our medical team, wellness coach, friends, family, and spiritual advisors, and on this path, whether we realize it or not, we are going to need their support every step of the way. It is important to be proactive in the beginning of our caregiving journeys by creating our Inspired Caregiver Support Teams and making distribution lists. We can ask our families, friends, and spiritual advisors if they would like to become a part of our support teams when we are in great need. We'd be surprised how many of our loved ones want to help, but do not know how. By creating our teams, not only will they feel good about being able to help us, we can feel secure knowing friends and family have committed to helping when we need their support. One of the most efficient tools for communicating with family and friends is Facebook.* Not only can we keep abreast of family and friends who are on Facebook, but we can inform them all at once if we need assistance in any way.

Lisa and Gonzalo have been Inspired Caregivers since the birth of their daughter, Ysabel, who is thirteen years young. She was born with a rare metabolic disorder, which flung them into a life of hospital stays, doctors' visits, and constant observation of their daughter. Ysabel was in the hospital again, and this time, Lisa used Facebook as her distribution list to inform her friends and family.

"We didn't have the time to call and speak with everyone. Facebook was a great way to let everyone know about Ysabel's situation and update them, as well as request prayers. It was also a great way for me to release my frustrations about our stay and how tired I was," Lisa reminisces. "And when I had a chance, I could read people's posts back to me, which meant a lot, because they were all so encouraging. I didn't have to stop and take a phone call; phone calls are problematic in the hospital, and answering individual emails can be so time consuming."

Facebook is an excellent tool for getting our wants and needs out to our support teams.

"I wrote, 'Okay, we're finally going home. Is anyone up to making and bringing us a meal?' and friends and family members coordinated dinners for us when we finally returned home, without two families bringing dinner on the same evening. It was so needed and so nice."

In Lisa and Gonzalo's case, Facebook prevented friends from showing up at the hospital. "Scheduling a good time for a visit can be problematic. We may pick a time, but now the doctors and specialists are making their rounds, or the nurses are giving reports, or our food is coming. Trying to coordinate visits can become a pain. Plus, Ysabel's cranky and tired, and we're cranky and tired."

Unfortunately, there can be disadvantages to using Facebook. Some of us may become depressed on Facebook as we see others having exciting, eventful lives, and may feel stuck and tied to the heavy burden of responsibilities for which we never planned. Lisa understands this all too well. "We all go through this feeling, but we have to choose how we feel, and that's part of having a joyful heart—rejoicing with those who rejoice and mourning with those who mourn."

Have you created your Inspired Caregiver Support Team and a distribution list?
Would Facebook be an efficient tool for you to use?

_____

_____

_____

_____

_____

_____

There are people who care and support me.
I reach out and let my needs be known.

Facebook is the most used social networking service at the time of this book's printing.
Please see our reference page regarding Facebook.

Sing...Dance...Laugh... Love...Live!

"Sing like no one's listening, love like you've never been hurt, dance like nobody's watching, and live like it's heaven on earth."

~Mark Twain

Live your life aloud! Being a caregiver doesn't mean we should or need to diminish our joys for living. Living our lives, feeling all our emotions, and doing the things that make us happy add to the well-being of all whose lives we touch. Give yourself permission to stop working and serving others and take time for yourself at least once a week to restore and replenish your body and soul by:

Joining a spiritual/religious group

Taking a creative writing class

Joining a walking club

Watching funny movies via DVD or at the movie theater

Getting a massage, pedicure, and/or manicure

Participating in golf, bowling, tennis, swimming, kayaking, and other activities

Window-shopping

Walking or hiking in nature

Taking a yoga, meditation, and/or a stress relief class

Taking a dance class

Taking a cooking class

Learning a musical instrument

Going out to lunch with your friends

Reading a great book

Journaling

Attending inspirational and motivational workshops

Are you consistently taking time out for yourself to replenish your soul? If not, make a list of activities for you to start enjoying once a week.

_____

_____

_____

_____

_____

_____

I take time out for myself at least once a week. I embrace all my feelings. I am willing to try something new.

Warning to Caregivers Who Care Too Much

"Sometimes caring too much for others means you don't care enough for yourself."

~ Unknown

If you are a caregiver who has made the commitment and dedication to honor yourself by taking time out for your mental, physical, spiritual, and emotional health every week, whatever you do, do not carry the responsibility for others. In other words, if you are a member of a dance group or spiritual study group, and one of the members wants you to cook the meal for a special gathering, or someone confides that he or she needs help that will take much of your time and energy, *it is best to decline.* It is important for you to remember that you are participating in these groups as a personal retreat, to receive nourishment and joy, not to add more responsibility.

If we make carrying the burden of responsibility a habit because we have caring hearts and have endured during times of crisis, we will be viewed as dependable, proactive, and solution-oriented. Others will sense this, and we will become the pillar for everyone. Like the loved ones we care for, others will become dependent upon our strength and lean more and more on us.

When asked to carry more responsibility, it is best to respond gently by saying, "I would love to, but this is not a good time for me. I'm sure there's someone in our group who can help with this." To prevent this situation from occurring in the first place, we may want to discuss boundaries and limitations with our class/group leaders in the beginning, explaining that we joined the group for rejuvenation and healing and cannot accept any more responsibility at this time.

If we feel guilty protecting our time and energy by saying no, a self preserving word for us, our wellness coaches (*later discussed in "Therapy: The New Black"*) can help us. Saying yes to unnecessary responsibility may be hazardous to our health and the health of our loved ones.

Do you have a hard time saying no to the demands and requests around you? Have you added more responsibility to your plate than necessary? Are the activities you agreed to do synergistic to your goal of being an Inspired Caregiver? If not, how can you release some of that responsibility to someone else?

_____

_____

_____

_____

_____

_____

When I say no to others I am saying yes to me!
The greatest gift I can offer to those I love and care
for is the gift of taking care of me.

Don't Do Guilt

"I must learn to love the fool in me, the one who feels too much, talks too much, takes too many chances, wins sometimes and loses often, lacks self-control, loves and hates, hurts and gets hurt, promises and breaks promises, laughs and cries."

~Theodore Isaac Rubin

Guilt is the rot of the caregiver's soul! We could have done more. We should be better organized. We should have more energy. We shouldn't become impatient. We should be more compassionate and understanding. We should not feel so much resentment and anger. We should be able to keep up with all the medical bills. We should be better caregivers. Should of, could of, would of.

Some of us feel a deep, piercing pain of guilt shadowing our souls because we have lost our tempers and lashed out with ugly words or raised a hand to our loved ones out of sheer frustration while in overwhelm. Some of us feel guilty because we secretly wish for our loved ones to pass away soon as their care has become a great cross to bear. Perhaps some of us have promised never to place our loved ones in a "home," only to revoke that promise when the care became too great.

Regardless of what we feel guilty about, it is imperative we let that guilt go. Women, especially, feel this guilt, as women have been conditioned in many societies to place their families' needs before their own. They are frowned upon and considered selfish if they place their own needs first. By discussing our feelings honestly with an inspired wellness coach and/or caregivers' support group, we discover we are not the only caregivers with these feelings and find tools and support to help release this unnecessary and destructive emotion.

Are you experiencing guilt while caring for your loved one? If so, where will you go to release this emotion?

_____

_____

_____

_____

_____

_____

_____

Each day I do the best I can. I am guilt free.
I am enough.

Protect and Control Your Time and Money

"You must master your time rather than becoming a slave to the constant flow of events and demands on your time. And you must organize your life to achieve balance, harmony, and inner peace."

~ Brian Tracy

The path of the caregiver can be extremely turbulent. If we do not protect and control our time, we may become like a feather in the wind, twirling at every demand and appointment. If we constantly leave our businesses or jobs to attend doctors' appointments during peak financial hours, not only will we lose money, we may eventually lose our businesses or jobs, as well.

When the receptionist makes appointments for our loved ones, unless it is an emergency, we must claim a time that is best for us. We cannot afford to be bullied into accepting a time that does not work for us. If the appointments are ongoing, such as physical therapy appointments, we should schedule our preferred times weeks in advance to secure our appointed time/dates. For example, if we are required to take our loved ones twice a week to physical therapy, and after four p.m. on Tuesdays and Thursdays are the best times for us, we should immediately set our appointments for these times and dates six to eight weeks in advance. If our preferred hours are not available, perhaps we can arrange with our employers or business partners to make up the hours lost to appointments. Remember, we want the appointments to work for us, not against us. Time is money and energy, so we should be mindful in protecting ours.

Are you allowing appointments to control you instead of you controlling them? If so, how can you make your loved one's appointments work for you?

_____

_____

_____

I make appointments work for my schedule and manage my money wisely and with ease.

Laughter is the Key to Good Health and Happiness

"At the height of laughter, the universe is flung into a kaleidoscope of new possibilities."

~Jean Houston

Have you ever laughed so hard, so loud, and so long, that tears actually leaked down your cheeks while you struggled to catch your breath? If you can't remember the last time you did, then it is a good time to make laughter one of your priorities. An easy way to obtain this laughter is to participate in laughter yoga, founded by Dr. Maden Kataria (Laughter Clubs International). In laughter yoga, large groups of people gather to laugh aloud together. The laughter is forced in the beginning, and it grows into belts of uncontrolled laughter and joy! According to Dr. Maden Kataria, fake laughter brings the same benefits as real laughter, benefits that include building our immune systems and releasing stress. For more information, search under "laughter yoga" at youtube.com and watch people practice this fun and infectious yoga all over the world.

~ SOMETIMES LAUGHTER IS THE BEST MEDICINE~

TIA'S STORY

I remember attending a laughter yoga class after an unusually trying day. I almost didn't go, because I was exhausted and a little disappointed about an interaction with a colleague. The fact that the instructor was a friend gave me extra incentive and so I decided to go.

At first, it felt silly, and the laugh was forced and fake. After a while and a few snorting sounds—whining, wheezing trailers to the laughter—I was in full-blown deep belly laughter, and the tears of joy started flowing. I laughed so hard my stomach was tight. I left with my vibration completely raised and could not identify what I was disappointed about when I initially came to class.

Below are other ways to bring laughter into your life, and the life of your loved one, as well:

- Watch a funny movie at least once a week.

- Watch an episode of your favorite sitcom once a day.

- Listen to comedians via audio CD while cleaning your home, cooking, or driving.

- Go to youtube.com and watch your favorite comedians or find new ones, at no charge!

- Read comic strips and joke books.

A fun game to play is to write down (or audio record) all of the things that were said, written, or that happened during your day that made you smile or giggle. (There is plenty of material if children surround you.) Soon you will have created your own personalized comedy book that you can read (or listen to) when you need a lift.

Most of us have heard of patients curing their cancer through laughter therapy: laughing for hours on a daily basis by watching comedy movies and sitcoms. If there are any truths to these claims, then why wouldn't every human being make laughter a priority? We do know that at the very least, laughter makes us feel good.

Are you laughing on a daily basis? If not, how can you add more laughter to your life?

_____

_____

_____

_____

_____

_____

I love to watch funny movies and look for humor in all situations!
Every day is filled with great laughter!

Boundaries

"The purpose of having boundaries is to protect and take care of ourselves."

~ Robert Burney

"Boundary: Something that indicates bounds or limits"
Random House *Webster's Dictionary*

Many of us follow the commandment "Love one another." When it relates to caregiving, it is important to love one another with boundaries. We must acknowledge that we are included in "love one another." We need to love and nourish ourselves to freely love our loved ones without resentment and overwhelm. Many times our loved ones become accustomed to being served every day. They have entire teams of people at their beck and call, and we, their caregivers, play the roles of:

- Entertainer
- Support team
- Cook
- Maid
- Counselor
- Chauffer
- Personal assistant
- Nurse

Our loved ones' health and well-being are the center of their universe, and ours as well. As our loved ones' needs become less demanding and we begin to craft our schedules to meet our needs, our loved ones may feel our withdrawal and panic, demanding more of our time. Our loved ones may tempt us to watch movies when they know we have planned to walk with a friend or spend time working on a project we are excited about. This is when tough love and discipline is essential for survival.

Loved ones may intentionally or unintentionally attempt to make us feel guilty or even have a temper tantrum when we refuse to surrender and accept their invitations or demands. When this happens, it is important that we keep our commitments to ourselves. If we do not, feelings of resentment and regret may seep into our beings and dampen our caregiving skills.

Wellness coach Donna L. Wood, a licensed psychotherapist practicing in Santa Cruz, California and the San Francisco Bay Area, stresses the importance of setting boundaries in relationships. She states, "When enforcing our boundaries, first and foremost, we are caring for ourselves, but we are also helping others to have a clear understanding of what we consider *acceptable* behavior. We are reflecting back to them what is *not acceptable* and, therefore, providing them an opportunity to consider that information and *make necessary changes*. If we ignore the behavior or accept the behavior, not only are we undermining ourselves, but we are denying the other person an opportunity to learn about themselves and to grow, and ultimately, we deny them the opportunity for a healthy relationship with us." When urgent care is not needed, it is in the best interest of our loved ones to keep our commitments to ourselves.

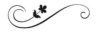

Are you slipping into the habit of surrendering to un-necessary demands and requests by your loved one during time you have scheduled for yourself? How can you prevent this from happening in the future?

_____

_____

_____

_____

_____

_____

By setting clear boundaries, I am taking care of me!

Therapy – The New Black!

Become Unstoppable with the Help of Your Wellness Coach!

"I love therapy! There's nothing like talking to someone who has no emotional tie to your life."

~Eva Mendes

Therapy is the new black, especially in Hollywood. More and more entertainers are obtaining balance with their wellness coaches. Caroline Rhea, actress and comedian, joked, "Being in therapy is great. I spend an hour just talking about myself. It's kind of like being the guy on the date."

When we are serious about becoming successful golfers or tennis players, or just becoming fit, we don't think twice about seeking coaches to guide us to greatness. Those desiring a successful business will seek a business coach. Now, life and dream coaches are the rave, helping us to not only survive in this world, but to live the lives about which we have only dreamed.

Obtaining an excellent wellness coach is essential to becoming an Inspired Caregiver and living a healthier life, especially if we are caring for parents with Alzheimer's or dementia. This is the time when buried childhood issues can resurface, causing great strife in our relationships with family members and ourselves, inhibiting our ability to give our best care.

Wellness coaches are professional licensed clinical psychologists, psychologists, psychotherapists, clinical social workers, psychiatrists, and mental health counselors who are passionate about their professions and the well-being of their clients. They are dedicated to coaching us to emotional and mental wellness and clarity. Many wellness coaches have become certified life coaches, as well.

One of the many reasons wellness coaches are so attractive is that they are sworn to confidentiality, forbidden to disclose their clients' identities or topics of discussion. This means we can release our pettiest and darkest thoughts and feelings, and they stay with them. What is said to the wellness coach stays with the wellness coach.* Wellness coaches use assertive, positive, and progressive techniques to help us through our caregiving journeys. They also help us process any negative events we have experienced that may subconsciously sabotage our success and happiness.

A negative experience can be traumatic events that happened to us or around us that made us fearful of moving forward in our lives and relationships. It can also refer to smaller events that we find ourselves talking and/or thinking about with anger, resentment, irritation, disappointment, shame, and/or grief. These experiences need to be processed safely and skillfully with our wellness coaches and released, so we can move forward to a healthier, happier future.

In Anita Moorjani's book, *Dying to Be Me*, Anita experienced a near-death experience as she was dying from cancer, in which she was shown that illnesses start on an energetic level before they become physical. This idea is synergistic to studies of how dis-ease can develop into disease if we do not return to our centers and live balanced lives.

If illness starts in our energies before it manifests physically, as stated in Anita Moorjani's book (and as is believed by many progressive wellness coaches and medical professionals), then having a wellness coach is imperative to our physical health, as well. If we feel disappointment, grief, resentment, shame, anger, rage, betrayal, irritation, frustration, hopelessness, and other negative, defeating emotions, it is a good indication that these emotions are starting to nest in our energies and can lead us to overwhelm and perhaps even manifest as a serious illness. An excellent wellness coach may not only guide us back to our centers, he or she just might save our lives.

Do you have a wellness coach passionately guiding you through your caregiving journey? If not, write down five areas in your life in which a wellness coach could help you. We encourage you to find the right one for you as soon as possible.

It is an act of self-love to seek a wellness coach to support me.

*Please see our reference page regarding exceptions to confidentiality.

Breathe

Inhale...exhale...breathe

"Breathing in, there is only the present moment. Breathing out, it is a wonderful moment."

~Thich Nhat Hanh

Just as our bodies crave water and nutrients, our souls crave silence. This silence is drowned out on a daily basis by negative images and suggestions on television and radio and in print. We are bombarded with negativity on televisions, which are now being placed in banks, hospitals, cars, grocery stores, and gas stations, as well as in our own homes. It is no wonder why many of us are experiencing anxiety, fear, worry, road rage, irritability, insomnia, and stomach upset. Our subconscious minds are assaulted with negative messages almost everywhere we go.

A beautiful way to obtain balance, peace-of-mind, and a healthy body is to practice the ancient art of meditation. Meditation quiets our minds and forces us to concentrate on only one thing, such as our breath, a sound, a word, a phrase, or an intention. Many meditation and breathing techniques, as well as visual and walking meditations, can be practiced. For some of us, meditation can be intimidating, leaving us wondering if we are doing it "right." Finding the meditation practice that works for each of us is key to incorporating this healthy stress reliever in our lives. If we have active minds that are hard to slow and quiet, a more active, guided meditation might be best for us by directing our thoughts with positive statements, such as, "There is enough time for me to do the things I am called to do."

By changing what we do every day without thought—breathing—we can greatly improve our well-being. We often hold our breath, tense our muscles, and breathe shallowly. When we are mindful of our breathing and breathe deeply, we can reduce our stress and improve our mental health. As we breathe deeply, the oxygen gives us energy and releases endorphins (the feel-good chemical in our brains). Think of taking time to breathe deeply as our natural happiness dosage. So, breathe deeply, and be happy. If it is easy for you to empty your mind and stay present in your meditation, use this time to appreciate all that you have. Being in gratitude as you meditate and breathe deeply can replenish your mind, body, and soul.

<u>In just ten to twenty quiet minutes a day, meditation can:</u>

- Improve concentration
- Enhance sexual attractiveness
- Release stress and anxiety
- Boost your immune system
- Slow the aging process
- Cool hot flashes
- Prevent sleep deprivation
- Increase performance and productivity

~*FEEL THE POWER OF YOUR BREATH*~

According to Thich Nhat Hanh, Buddhist monk, teacher, author, poet, and peace activist, life is available only in the present moment. Focusing on our breath helps us to be in the present. "Breathing in, I calm body and mind. Breathing out, I smile. Dwelling in the present moment, I know this is the only moment."

The breathing technique below, created by peak performance strategist and author, Anthony Robbins, from his personal achievement system, "Personal Power," is wonderful for helping you focus your attention on the moment and increasing the quality of your life, specifically your physical life and energy level:

Inhale through your nose and into your abdomen for
1 count
Hold for 4 counts
Exhale slowly from your abdomen for 2 counts

For example: Gently inhale for 3 counts, expanding your abdomen with air, then hold your breath for 12 counts, and then slowly release your breath for 6 counts, noticing the fall of your abdomen as you exhale. When this becomes comfortable for you, increase your starting breath count to 4 counts, and then 5 counts, and so on.

Whether you desire to reduce stress by dwelling in the present moment or by obtaining better physical health and more energy, Anthony Robbins' Power Breathing is a wonderful technique to include in your daily practice or anytime you feel stressed. For the best results, it is suggested to do this in sets of ten deep breaths, three times a day.

www.TonyRobbins.com
Used with permission. © Robbins Research International, Inc.

Have you found a meditation/breathing practice that works well for you? Feel free to write that practice

below as a commitment to your self-care. If not, are you willing to search the internet for a meditation technique that works best for you? Once you have found a technique, record it below.

_____

_____

_____

_____

_____

_____

With each breath, I release stress and inhale strength.

Don't Worry, Be Happy

"Worrying is like a rocking chair. It gives you something to do, but gets you nowhere."

~Glenn Turner

Sometimes in the midst of our caregiving, anxious thoughts may flood our minds, "What if my loved one runs out of money? What if I do? What if I lose my job? I'm tired; how am I going to continue living this way? Who can help me with all of this? What do I do next? What if I get sick? Where is God? These are all important questions, which your Inspired Caregiving Team can help you solve. But what about the nagging questions and fears that are out of your control? How do you handle anxiety?

When these heart racing, blood pressure spiking moments erupt, a great exercise is to sit down calmly and list all of the challenging situations you have faced in your life. Write down not only the situations, but also all of your worries and concerns that stormed your mind at that time. Now, with hindsight, write down what actually happened. You may discover that during those times of uncertainty, solutions appeared almost miraculously, and your problems were solved. Perhaps some of the obstacles were actually blessings in disguise, for the outcome was far more beneficial than you could have possibly imagined. Carry this list with you to help ease your discomfort should you have another panic attack. By reading this list and releasing your worries to your higher power, you will gently be lifted back to center again.

Another way to tame your mind when it starts to go into worry mode is to capture what you are worrying about and follow the train of thought to the "worst-case" scenario. If you ask the question, "And then what?" repeatedly, until you can't go any further, you might be surprised. You may discover that in the worst-case scenario, the very thing you feared most isn't the end of the world, and there are no problems that can't be overcome or that we can't live through. Think of all the things you have ever worried about. Did the energy and time spent worrying about those perceived problems really make a difference? Probably not.

Do you habitually worry or experience panic attacks?
What effective tool or tools can you use to bring you
back to center?

_____

_____

_____

_____

_____

_____

Worry is misspent energy. I focus on what I can do. I am capable, willing, and able.

Exercise Three Times a Week!

"I'd do anything for a body like hers, except for diet and exercise."

~ Unknown

Have you ever noticed that when we walk or exercise, we feel better? Our minds are sharper and we have an abundance of energy. "I feel great," we tell ourselves. "I love this feeling! I must do this every single day!" So, why do we stop? The hard, cold fact is that we haven't made exercise a habit, and therefore, we haven't made our physical health a priority.

Time after time, studies show that if we just do some simple exercises three times a week, the benefits are amazing. Below are a few:

- Increases energy
- Improves memory
- Improves self-esteem
- Promotes quality rest
- Helps ward off depression
- Slows the effects of aging
- Reduces joint pain
- Reduces risks of illnesses, such as cardiovascular disease, diabetes, and cancer
- Promotes a healthier, leaner body
- Increases productivity

Although there are no guarantees, we must take care of ourselves now so others won't need to later. We must train consistently, as if we are professional athletes, because we are! Our bodies need to endure the demands and sometimes-toxic environments we tread day after day after day.

Consider customizing a simple exercise program with your medical doctor in conjunction with a physical therapist and/or fitness trainer to create the most effective plan with the time available to you. Your plan should include techniques to overcome your weaknesses. For example, if you have a history of not following through with commitments to yourself, consider having a friend exercise with you consistently as an accountability buddy. If you are not able to exercise for the entire twenty minutes, perhaps you should break the twenty minutes into two ten-minute workouts, such as a brief ten-minute walk in the morning and another one in the early evening.

To achieve the maximum benefit, make every exercise matter. Do your best when moving and be consistent. You will feel the improvement not only in your body and mind, but in your caregiving as well.

Have you made exercising twenty minutes a day, three times a week, a consistent habit in your life? If not, what steps are you willing to take to shift this healthy routine into your life?

_____

_____

_____

_____

I exercise for at least twenty minutes a day, three times a week, and I feel great!

Make Your Support Group Your Sanctuary

"Alone we can do so little; together we can do so much."

~Helen Keller

The journey of the caregiver can be a very lonely one. We may feel that our friends and family have withdrawn, leaving us isolated and alone. We may be so consumed with the health and well-being of our loved ones that we abandon our own needs and desires. We may even stop reaching out to our friends and family for help as we continue to carry this heavy burden alone. The truth is that we are not alone. It is important to find our hearts homes in strong support groups, preferably at the beginning of our journeys. This will prevent us from getting lost in the dense fog of illusion whispering lies that no one cares nor will they ever understand our situation.

By joining caregiver support groups once a week, we will discover that others feel the same way and that there are solutions to our tallest, steepest mountains. By talking to other caregivers about our deepest, darkest thoughts and feelings, we release the pent-up energy that causes sleepless nights, anxieties, and dis-ease. We not only prevent disease from manifesting, but we feel lighter, healthier, and happier.

If we cannot leave our homes, there are on-line care-giver support groups. Our medical teams may be able to help guide us to safe, supportive groups. If we prefer to join support groups for caregivers with loved ones suffering from specific illnesses, our medical teams may have that information, as well. We can always visit www. TheInspiredCaregiver.com for a list of potential support groups or search the Internet.

Are you attending a caregiver group on a weekly basis? Have you discovered a supportive caregiver chat line/ support group on-line? Is there a caregiver group in your area you can attend? If not, will you ask your medical team to help you find or create one?

_____

_____

_____

_____

_____

_____

I deserve to be supported, and others are there for me; all I need to do is ask. There is an abundance of support for me just for the asking.

Give Yourself Permission to Cry

Release that Pent-Up Energy!

"What soap is for the body, tears are for the soul."

~Jewish Proverb

Because we need to be pillars of strength for the ones we are caring for, it is easy to suppress our emotions to the point of numbness, irritability, and impatience. If we do not eventually acknowledge our negative emotions, it is only a matter of time before our bodies begin acknowledging them for us in the form of dis-ease. The question is not if our bodies will begin to break down. The question is when.

When we cry, we release our suppressed emotions, which help to prevent depression and dis-ease. Crying removes toxins from our bodies, helps to lubricate and clean our eyes, and has many other benefits. Crying is a natural, healthy process that we need to give ourselves permission to experience when the need arises. Caregivers can be very proud. We may not want to show signs of grief or weakness or confess when caregiving has become too much. The truth is that we all have weak, vulnerable moments, and sometimes during the dark nights of our soul, we have had enough. Feelings of defeat and hopelessness spill out without permission, causing great embarrassment, as it can happen anytime, anywhere, and in front of anyone.

One of the most effective and private places we can release grief and other disempowering emotions that partner with grief is in the shower. No one can hear us, and if we desire even more privacy, meaning, we just might have a wailing fest, we can have music playing in the background to help mask our howls.

When we step into the shower, we can allow the warm water to wash away our tears of frustration, disappointment, and betrayal, and just cry, cry, cry. Imagine the water turning gray as it rushes down the drain with all the negative energy released from our bodies. When we finally step out of our showers, we will feel exhausted and our eyes and faces may be swollen. We can dry off, snuggle into our favorite pajamas, and slip into clean, warm beds. We will most likely get the best rest we have had in months. In the weeks that follow, we will feel more patient, more loving and have solutions to some of our most troublesome problems. We will have been energetically cleansed and rejuvenated. It's a new day!

~*CLEANSING CRY AT THE OCEAN'S EDGE*~

One very late afternoon, Tia and I decided to park her car along the side of a cliff and talk privately while sipping our tea and watching the violent waves crash against the rocks. It had been a turbulent year for both of us and the ocean seemed to speak our silence. As we shared our worries, two women pulled up next to us. One petite woman got out of the passenger seat and rushed towards the ocean. She started screaming and raising her arms in the air, as if cursing it. She screamed and screamed as the waves helped to muzzle the sound. Tia and I froze, concerned that she was going to take her own life, and we watched intensely, ready to call 911 from our cell phones.

The woman's screams flowed into a deep, haunting, hollow sob from a place we seldom go. Tia and I couldn't help but silently sob with her. Empathy and perspective enveloped us. We thought our troubles were tormenting, but did they really compare to the horror this woman felt? Had she lost her husband? Her child?

In that moment, we realized what was important in life. No matter what disappointments we suffer, none of it truly matters except our health and the health and well-being of the ones we love!

We asked the driver if we could be of assistance, but she politely replied that her friend needed to mourn. There was nothing any of us could do.

Julia Cameron, author of *The Sound of Paper,* states, "All life contains great blows from which we must recover." Whether we mourn the delay of our dreams in order to care for another or lose our homes or businesses, a loved one, or how a loved one used to be, we can release our sorrows under the sound of crashing waves or the mask of steaming showers. These are great ways to allow ourselves to mourn as all of our emotions are washed away. Allow your tears to heal, cleanse, and release the burden that sometimes comes when we are called to care for another.

In which ways can you safely release your tears?

_____

_____

_____

Tears are a sign of my strength. I care deeply and celebrate the healing of each teardrop.

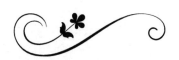

Caregiver Abuse ~ When You Are on the Receiving End of Abuse

"Sometimes the patients are dealing with their own pain so much that it clouds their judgment."

~ Sheila Shaw

Sometimes our loved ones are difficult and/or abusive. It is important *that if we choose to continue to care for them*, we love them with detachment. We are not the cause of their pain and unhappiness. It is not our fault that they are ill or disabled. Sometimes we can do everything possible to make them happy and they will still be unhappy. Sometimes they choose to be unhappy. It may be their habitual manner or a manipulative tool. By maintaining our happiness and health, even if our loved ones are unhealthy or unhappy, we ensure our ability to go the long haul.

Some of us may be caring for loved ones who suffer from narcissistic personality disorder or another type of personality disorder. Personality disorders can prevent them from appreciating and recognizing our unconditional love and care. For our own well-being, we must recognize this in our loved ones' cases. We can find information on personality disorders in bookstores, libraries, youtube. com (video information), and Internet websites. We may find it helpful to consult with our wellness coaches regarding this matter, as well. It is self-preservation and easier to love a difficult person with detachment, and therefore, easier to take nothing they say or do against us personally.

Our loved ones may be difficult due to the effects of the medications they are taking. We should immediately explore this possibility with their medical teams.

If our loved ones do not have a personality disorder and their difficulty is not due to their medications, we can speak to them about how they can help us. If they continue to be abusive and difficult, perhaps we can speak to their medical teams about referring us to great support groups and/or wellness coaches *(if we do not have one yet)*. In these groups and sessions, our voices will be embraced and heard with understanding, so that gentle healing and compassion can begin.

If our loved ones will not participate in therapy of any kind, and *we continue to choose to care for them*, it is imperative that we love with detachment, and make our health THE priority, as we will need an extremely strong immune system and armor to withstand the continual abuse.

~ REAL WORLD EXAMPLE ~
PEGGI'S STORY

I spoke to Ida, who was caring for her demanding and manipulative mother. Every time Ida tried to grab a break to walk or do something healthy for herself, her mother fell down on purpose or acted as if she felt weak and sick. She would not allow Ida to leave her side and wanted Ida to do everything for her, including organizing her medications, which she was quite capable of doing herself. She used harsh words to make her feel guilty. When Ida left to go grocery shopping, she would call her daughter to watch her mother. However, her mother was independent and did everything for herself whenever her granddaughter was around. Once Ida returned and her daughter left, Ida's mother, once again, played helpless.

When we spoke, Ida was sobbing tears of hopeless frustration. She did not want to disrespect her mother. However, she had just returned from a doctor's appointment and had been warned that her blood pressure and cholesterol were alarmingly high. The doctor strongly urged her to exercise consistently, manage her stress levels, and eat healthier foods. Ida could not see how to do this, as her mother would not allow it.

After listening for almost an hour, I determined Ida had far surpassed overwhelm, and I offered her some of the tips in this book, including exploring co-dependency issues with a wellness coach. I shared my opinion that if she chose not to make her health a priority, someone else may have to care for her mother, perhaps her daughter. Ida would not be around. This was the bottom line, and it was time Ida did what she needed to do for her own health and well-being, despite how her mother felt about it. The choice was up to Ida.

To be an Inspired Caregiver, we must love our loved ones through their pain, but with boundaries and detachment. It is extremely important not to stay too long in an environment that is toxic to our health (mentally, physically, spiritually, and emotionally). The consequences can be fatal.

Is the person you are caring for difficult or abusive? If so, in what ways is he or she abusive, and what steps can you take now to create a healthy, cooperative relationship?

_____

_____

_____

_____

_____

_____

I am love. I draw on that truth when challenged. Everyone is doing the best they know how. All is well. I show love and compassion for myself and those I care for.

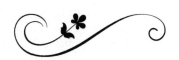

Nutrition! No Ifs, Ands, or Buts. It's a Must!

"Today, more than 95% of all chronic disease is caused by food choice, toxic food ingredients, nutritional deficiencies, and lack of physical exercise."

~ Mike Adams

In our society, there is a misconception about what a "healthy" body looks like. Quite often, someone in a "normal" weight range suffers from malnutrition. Regardless of our current weight, we may not be receiving the proper nutrients we need for sustained energy and brain efficiency. A malnourished caregiver can experience heightened irritability, fatigue, forgetfulness, and the dreaded overwhelm. Fueling our bodies with healthy foods, such as vegetables, fruit, and legumes (preferably organic), and decreasing our intake of meat, dairy, and processed foods is part of being Inspired Caregivers. Not only do we look healthier, we feel healthier.

When shifting to healthier foods, it is important to be mindful of how we feel after each meal and snack. Does this meal make us feel tired, or do we have more energy? Are we experiencing headaches, irritability, digestion upset, or shakiness after each meal? If so, could we be suffering from growing and often misdiagnosed gluten and dairy intolerances? Limiting our alcohol, sodas, sugar, and coffee intake and increasing our water intake (preferably filtered) will help us to perform better, as well.

<u>Little shifts we can make to promote healthier eating are:</u>

- Never go shopping when hungry, as we may purchase fatty, unhealthy foods and spend above our budgets.

- Prepare grab-n-go snacks, such as boiled eggs, apples, almonds, walnuts, and/or sticks of carrots and celery, or pre-made half-sandwiches filled with vegetables, egg, hummus, and/or our favorite sandwich meats.

- Never eat when on the telephone or watching TV, as we need to be mindful of what nutrition we are placing into our bodies at all times.

- Portion out our food to promote mindfulness of the amounts we are eating.

- Juicing is an excellent option for adding healthy nutrients into our bodies between meals. Some juicing combinations pack more nutrients than many traditional full meals.

- Making smoothies, such as organic apple, carrot, orange smoothies and spinach, yam, apple, carrot smoothies, can be a quick meal or snack filled with vitamins, minerals, and antioxidants and we get fiber, as well! One of our favorite books on quick, nutritious smoothies is *The Everything Green Smoothies Book* by Britt Brandon with Lorena Novak Bull. This simple, easy-to-read book includes 300 nutritious smoothie recipes, and it is filled with great nutritional information and tips.

- If juicing or smoothies are not for you, purchase a large basket, and at the start of your week, fill it with organic apples, oranges, and bananas. Make it a goal to eat all the fruit by the end of every week. By doing this, you feed your body healthy nutrients you may not have otherwise eaten.*

- To promote drinking more water, try filling a nice, colorful glass bottle with filtered water and pour the water into a wine glass. Psychologically, the water may be easier to drink, and we will drink more of it, as opposed to drinking from a plain glass. The clinking of the glass and the sound of the water gently splashing into the wine glass can be therapeutic and give us a sense of calm and peace.

- We can consider customizing a simple nutritional plan with our medical doctors, in conjunction with nutritionists, to create the most effective plans for our bodies with the time and funds we have available.

~*RECLAIM YOUR MEAL TIMES*~

Remember when a meal was more than a function to satisfy our hunger? Reclaim meal times as an opportunity to sit and replenish your body and soul. Take the time to schedule a meal with a friend and enjoy the meal, drink, conversation, and moments together. Deciding to skip the fast food or rushed meal to eat at a more leisurely pace honors you and all that you do for others. Small touches, such as lighting a candle, pulling out a colorful tablecloth or placemats, and using dishes or glasses you love can make an everyday necessity a sacred time. So, schedule in that hour to fully enjoy a meal. You deserve it!

By making our health a priority, we make our loved ones our priorities. We cannot afford not to eat nutritious foods daily. Our loved ones depend on our well-being for their well-being.

Are you getting the proper nutrition you need to perform at your best? If not, what small shifts can you make in your eating habits to ensure this?

_____

_____

_____

_____

_____

_____

I love to eat healthy, nutritious foods that fuel my body with the vitamins and minerals it needs every day!

Consult with your medical team before juicing and adding more fruit to your diet if you are diabetic or suspect blood sugar issues.

Forgiveness

"To forgive is to set a prisoner free and discover that the prisoner was you."

~ Lewis Smedes

Many of us are the walking wounded, having emotional wounds we have carried alone for years, suppressing anger, shame, betrayal, depression and/or resentment towards specific individuals or circumstances. This pain can become heavier and resurface when triggered under the responsibility of caregiving, pushing us into overwhelm. Some of us are waiting for individuals to need our care, so we can repay them for the suffering endured while we were under their care. Some of us are harboring such deep pain inside we wait patiently for this day to come.

In either case, in order to free ourselves from the anchor that may be deep seated in the shadows within us, we must give ourselves permission to forgive and let it all go. Forgiving does not mean that we continue to place ourselves in an abusive situation nor are we agreeing with them. It does not mean we must communicate with the person or persons who hurt us. Forgiving is for our benefit emotionally, spiritually, physically, and mentally. When we truly forgive, we break the chains that bind us and begin to discover who we truly are: beautiful, loving, gifted, powerful individuals with endless possibilities.

Sometimes we have forgiven everyone in our lives except ourselves. Sometimes we are the most difficult people to forgive. We must learn to look at ourselves through the lens of love, compassion, and understanding. We strive to keep our balance through nutrition, rest, water, exercise, and sometimes medication, but we are only human and we make mistakes. We may subconsciously be angry with ourselves for losing our tempers or saying words to a loved one that we cannot take back. By not forgiving ourselves, we can spiral into feelings of unworthiness and depression.

Forgiveness is a process of releasing all the behaviors and events that do not define or honor us anymore. In order to release our wounds, we must release the negative energy that stews or rages silently within. Using the techniques discussed in the Anger Release chapter, the ocean and shower techniques, journaling, and writing letters to the person or persons who have offended us (without sending the letter) can help us through this process. We must release all of this energy, no holding back;

release any feelings of powerlessness, unworthiness, injustice, and betrayal. Give all of this energy to your higher power and pray to be released from it forever.

We suggest going through this process with a wellness couch as it is safe and confidential and forgiveness may be obtained faster and more thoroughly. Participating in retreats and workshops that specialize in releasing unforgiveness can be life defining, as well, and remind us that we are not alone in this process.

~*FORGIVENESS EXERCISE*~

There is a heavy cost to holding onto resentment and refusing to release and forgive those you feel have harmed you. If you think you do not need to forgive, try this exercise.

1. Buy a ten-pound bag of potatoes.
2. Take one potato for each word that completes the thought you have about the person you need to forgive and put it into a sack. Example: Thoughts: "He treated me poorly. He didn't support me. He is self-centered."
3. Now take that sack with you everywhere you go for the entire day. Notice the energy necessary just to carry your sack. This weight is similar to the weight you carry by not forgiving those who have harmed you.

For a healthy way to release this weight and experience the freedom of forgiveness, try this process:

1. Visualize the person you want to forgive. See a smile on his or her face. The person is happy to see you. You are also smiling and at ease in his or her presence. Breathe into that feeling.

2. Clearly and gently state what you feel the person did to hurt you or cause you pain. You may write this down if that feels more satisfying to you.

3. Imagine the person as a little child saying to you, "I did the best I knew how in the moment. You didn't deserve to be hurt, and I'm so sorry."

4. State the person's name and the following statement: _____, I forgive you completely and fully. This is not mine, and I release it. I am totally free and so are you.

I am grateful that I love myself enough to forgive and be free.

When we forgive those who trespass against us, we will have more energy, more compassion, and most importantly, more peace within our souls. We are happier and healthier, and all is well.

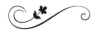

When you look back on your life's journey, is there someone you need to forgive? What steps will you take to begin this process?

_____

_____

_____

_____

_____

_____

I forgive those who have harmed me in any way. Today is a new day, and I have left all grudges in the past. My heart holds love, and all is well.

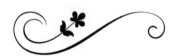

Sacred Rest

"Take rest; a field that has rested gives a bountiful crop."

~ Ovid

To keep balanced, we must never underestimate the power of rest. <u>Rest helps prevent</u>:

- Weight gain
- Difficulty in concentration
- Memory loss
- Irritability
- Impaired cognition
- Diabetes
- Heart problems
- Depression

- Impatience
- Automobile accidents
- Divorce
- Overwhelm

When we have had enough rest, we feel better, we communicate better, we think better, and our skin even looks better. Rest is sacred. It repairs our cells and nourishes, heals, and restores us to our center. Without it, we do not receive the healing we need to function at our best. It is imperative that we make rest the foundation of our self-care by obtaining seven to nine hours of quality sleep every evening. Some of the best ways to obtain sacred rest:

- Go to bed at the same time every evening and wake up at the same time every morning.

- Read something peaceful and comforting that nourishes our spirits before sleeping, such as *Sabbath*, by Wayne Muller.

- Do not watch television before sleeping, especially the news.

- Before retiring for the evening, clean the dishes or any area in our living spaces that cause us great restlessness, knowing we are waking up to it in the morning.

- Ask our nutritionists and/or holistic practitioners about vitamins, amino acids, minerals, herbs, and teas that will help us sleep.

- Transform our rooms with scents of lavender and block out lights or noise that discourage sleep.

- Exercising during our waking hours will help us sleep during sleeping hours.

- Limit our caffeine intake during the day, especially in the evening.

- Pray and give all of our worries to our higher power.

If our sleep is continuously broken by the needs of our loved ones, perhaps we can share shifts for night care with someone in the household. We can also have someone watch our loved ones during the day while we take a much-needed nap. We need to surrender ourselves to healing and sacred rest every night. We are worth it.

Do you get enough consistent rest nightly? If not, why not, and what nurturing practices can you put into place to ensure a good night's sleep?

_____

_____

_____

_____

_____

_____

When I rest, I have more to give to others and myself. I listen to my body and rest when needed. Resting is my time to relax, unwind, and rejuvenate. I feel good!

The Rewards of Caregiving

"The person who risks nothing, does nothing, has nothing, is nothing, and becomes nothing. He may avoid suffering and sorrow, but he simply cannot learn and feel and change and grow and love and live."

~Leo Buscaglia

Peggi's Caregiving Gift:

Caring for Rose was the most challenging time of my life. It pushed every part of me to the brink of destruction, and my thoughts wandered to dark, numbing places I never knew existed. However, when I look back at the time I cared for her, it was also a life defining time. What I discovered in the ruin of despair was indeed a treasure, and I am forever changed.

Rose and I used to sing in the car together. We laughed, and many times, she said something so hilarious I immediately wrote it down. For example, one day Rose was enjoying a Kit Kat (her favorite candy bar), and she looked at me and said, "Peggi, if I get to where I can't talk anymore, and you see me putting my hand up to my mouth like this [she tapped her hand on her mouth rapidly while looking at me with wide-open eyes], it means, 'Stick a Kit Kat in my mouth!'"

Rose and I savored our cappuccinos and enjoyed our shopping adventures. We enjoyed being together, just be-ing. I experienced what it was like to love and give without reward, and I discovered and rediscovered the treasure in Mother Teresa's work and others whose work and words gave me great peace and strength, such as Rumi, Jesus, Buddha, Maya Angelo, and Thich Nhat Hanh. Through the gift of caregiving, I learned that I must take care of myself, and that I am responsible for my health and happiness.

Not only did I learn to love more purely, I learned that what truly matters are not things. We cannot take them with us, and they are useless to us when we are sick. The most important investments we can make are in our own health and growth and in each other. Most of all, I learned more about me—how I react in times of crisis, how long I can endure, what I can withstand and no longer withstand, how my body and emotions are connected, and how they respond to stress. I discovered that my health matters. My life matters. I matter!

~TIA'S CAREGIVING GIFT~

When I received the news that required me to draw on strength I didn't know I had, it ended up being a gift in disguise. I had already lost my mother in my twenties, but then I received the call – my father needed a heart valve replaced immediately. I needed to care for my father after surgery and prepare for him to stay at my home with my family.

My dad was a renaissance man, an entrepreneur, a fiercely independent free spirit. He took great pride in helping others and was active and healthy. To need my help and care was very humbling for him. It was an adjustment for me to see my father as fragile and dependent on me for care while recovering from surgery. As I reflect on that time, I appreciate the vulnerability, trust, and surrender necessary for him to acknowledge he needed my care.

During the weeks of caregiving, something magical happened. I had a gift of a multi generational experience: grandpa was privy to the daily lives of his grandsons, and he had many opportunities to bond with them in an entirely new way. I was able to allow a very proud and independent father to soften into receiving love and care. This richness deepened our family bond.

In what way has your caregiving experience been a gift to you?

_____

_____

_____

_____

_____

_____

Today I look for the gifts that I have been given by taking care of others. I am better for this journey.

An Aha! Moment

Do You Know Who Will Take Care of You Should You Need Care?

"A loving heart is the truest wisdom."

~Charles Dickens

Rose was always a bit jealous of my other friends, as she was a possessive friend. When Rose had a stroke, our friend Sheila volunteered to help me care for her. Sheila bathed Rose and helped take care of Rose's two cats. Rose learned to see Sheila no longer as a threat to our friendship, but as another "sister." Rose grew in love. Rose often looked at me in bewilderment while I served her dinner or helped her with her physical therapy and said, "How did I know that the girl I met thirty years ago would be the one taking care of me now?"

While caring for Rose, we had an AHA discovery! Never in her wildest dreams would Rose have imagined that the young girl she met while vacationing with her husband in Hawaii and the young girl's friend, a person Rose disliked and rejected due to her own jealousy and insecurity, would lovingly care for her years later, during the most vulnerable time of her life.

The phrase "Love one another" is so wise. By loving one another, we invest in each other and in ourselves. Perhaps someday, when we need someone to care for us, it may not come from the person we expect, but from the person we *least* expect. It may be our sons or daughters-in-laws, our neighbors, friends, cousins, stepchildren, or stepparents whose love for us has assigned them to the honorable, yet dangerous position of caregiver.

Is there someone in your family or circle of friends who you have been rejecting due to prejudice, disapproval, insecurities, or jealousies? Take a soul journey and release all of your judgments to your higher power, and choose to love and accept them just the way they are.

_____

_____

_____

_____

_____

_____

I treat everyone with love and kindness. I am grateful for the people in my life who care about my well-being.

What Do You Mean You Don't Have Time?

"To achieve great things, two things are needed: a plan, and not quite enough time."

~Leonard Bernstein

When caregivers are confronted with "Are you taking time out for yourself on a weekly basis?" or "Are you taking twenty-minute breaks three times a week to exercise?" the most common answer we hear with clenched teeth is, "I don't have the time."

This may be the case in many situations; however, many of us have the time to watch TV a few hours a day and talk habitually on the telephone too long about matters that are not positive or healing. Many of us even make it a priority to watch the news three times a day, which feeds our subconscious minds with great fear and worry, intensifying our already stressed feelings.

If we are mindful of what activities dominate our time, we may discover we have an abundance of time to make our mental, physical, emotional, and spiritual health a priority. The real question is, "Are we willing to give up something we feel is good for something better for us?" If we enjoy watching the news three times daily, perhaps we can make a little shift. Instead of watching the morning news, we can take a brisk walk or sit out in the garden and bask in the beauty and fragrance of the flowers. While watching our favorite TV shows, we can jump on a mini-trampoline, ride a stationary bike, get on the treadmill, do sit-ups, pushups, leg lifts, stretches, or something that will improve our physical health and release pent-up energy.

By being mindful of how we spend our time and making the tiny shifts necessary to put our well-being first on our list of priorities, we can reclaim our lives and fill it with inspiration and good health. We're worth it!

Are you willing to evaluate the use of your time on a daily basis? What activities do you do that no longer serve you, and how can you replace these activities with something healthier for your body, mind, and soul?

_____

_____

_____

_____

_____

_____

Time is a valuable asset, and I use it wisely. There is always enough time for me.

Are You in Overwhelm?

Evaluate Where You Are Emotionally

"If I didn't do something, it was either going to be suicide or homicide!"

~Caregiver in overwhelm, before placing
his father in an assisted living facility

If you are:

- Depressed
- Frustrated
- Angry
- Resentful
- Irritable

- Fatigued

- Eating too much or too little

- Sleeping too much or too little

- Feeling as though your life doesn't belong to you anymore

- Feeling alone in your caregiving responsibilities

- Feeling completely depleted

- Feeling a sense of hopelessness

- Experiencing a loss of interest in the activities, people, and things that used to inspire you

- Thinking of hurting yourself and/or your loved one

…you may be in overwhelm.

If you answered yes to two or more of the questions above, please inhale, sit back, and create a plan to return to center. This is a very good indication you are in overwhelm. Overwhelm is another term for caregiver burnout, and once we are in overwhelm, it is very difficult to return to a healthy, positive state while continuing to care for your loved one.

If thoughts of hurting yourself and/or your loved one stream through your mind, run— don't walk—and find a wellness coach to provide the support you need to lift your burden. If you are thinking these thoughts while sinking deeply into the state of overwhelm, immediately call a 24-hour suicide crisis line or run to your local hospital. Most hospitals have a mental health department where someone will gently guide you to the care you need.

Sometimes we may not recognize that we are in overwhelm, because caregivers routinely mask our emotions. Many of us have been giving care to our loved ones for so many years we have forgotten what healthy emotions are.

~*A Moment in Overwhelm*~
Peggi's Story

I left Rose with a dear friend while I ran a few errands. As I drove, loneliness swept over me. In that moment, I needed to hear a comforting voice, so I called my sister, Kathleen. The first thing Kathleen asked was, "How are you doing with Rose?" She was very aware of all of the verbal abuse I was enduring; she had witnessed it several times. I laughed and replied, "Oh, Kathy, she's been so difficult and mean. Today I actually thought about taking her down Highway 1 and driving us both off the cliff. "What do you think of me now? AHHHAHAHHH!"

We both laughed hysterically at the absurdity of this vision, and then the phone went dead quiet for what seemed like forever. Kathleen's voice finally pierced the silence as she commanded, "That's great, Peg, but make sure YOU jump out of that car before it goes off the cliff!" Stunned by the serious tone, I quickly excused myself from the call. Tears flooded down my face. I abruptly pulled the car off the road and sobbed uncontrollably. Someone cared about me! Someone actually cared about MY well-being. In the chaos of my caregiving, I had forgotten this.

I was always taught to respect my elders and treat everyone with kindness. I gave Rose all my love and care. Abuse, however, starts with a thought. Although this homicidal thought was not one I seriously considered, it was a telltale sign that I was in overwhelm. It was time for me to reclaim my life and self worth by consulting with a wellness coach and Rose's medical team to create an exit plan.

It is important to be mindful of where we are emotionally at all times. If, after applying all of the tools in this book, we can no longer keep positive, inspired attitudes and give the best care to our loved ones and ourselves, we should immediately find trusted family members, friends, or assisted living facilities to care for them. We should prepare a caregiver's exit plan for our health and the health of our loved ones. No matter what criticism we receive from others, taking this much-needed step may not only prevent caregiver abuse, but save our own lives, as well.

Are you in overwhelm? If not, list what actions you can do to prevent caregiver overwhelm. If so, list what actions you must take immediately to bring yourself back to center.

_____

_____

_____

_____

_____

_____

I live a life of balance and recognize what serves me. I am at peace.

Resources at Your Fingertips

"Ask, and it shall be given you; seek, and ye shall find; knock, and it shall be opened unto you."

Matthew 7:7 King James Version

YouTube.com - A Great Resource, Empowerment, and Play Center!

If you seek, you may find it on YouTube.* YouTube.com is an excellent site on which to watch movies, comedy, old videos of favorite artists, and obtain tips on almost anything, including caregiving tips from caregivers and caregiving organizations. The world has become smaller, and we have great information at the touch of our fingertips.

If you are deep in the trenches of caregiving and feel drained and disempowered, when you have a few minutes, visit www.youtube.com. Enjoy watching motivational and spiritual videos by Anthony Robbins, Zig Ziglar, Joel Osteen, Les Brown, Dr. Wayne Dyer, Louise Hay, Loretta Laroche, or anyone with whom you resonate. In only five or ten minutes, it may create the surge of energy you need to feel refreshed, renewed, and recharged.

~POWER TIP~

Did you know that you could get the equivalent of a college education just by listening to books on CDs or MP3s? What if you used the time your loved one is resting or while you are at a doctor's appointment to expand your mind? Imagine what a positive effect it would have to listen to motivational and inspirational information during your drive time or while you are cleaning your home.

Amazon.com and other on-line bookstores can save time and money

There is something magical about a bookstore. We are surrounded by information we need to help with our caregiving and our own care. We may meet others who share our interests, spend a quiet moment in conversation with a friend, or be immersed in a book while sipping tea or coffee and enjoying a little treat at their coffee shop (if they have one). Sometimes bookstores have poetry readings and speaking events by authors, which can help us feel inspired again. Although we believe that on-line bookstores can never replace the exhilarating experience of actually spending time in one, many of us do not have the energy or time to do so.

This is when Amazon.com, barnesandnoble.com, or our favorite on-line bookstores can be wonderful tools for us. Many times, the books arrive in only a couple of days. With all the running around to hospitals, grocery stores, banks, physical therapy, and counseling sessions, this can be extremely helpful. It is always exciting to find a book, DVD, or CD in the mailbox to enjoy in the time we have designated for ourselves.

Do you have five minutes a day to watch or read information on the health and care of your loved one and yourself? Do you have access to material that makes you laugh and your heart sing? If not, write down a list of people who make you laugh and information you'd like to receive, and then allow your fingers to find this information on-line.

_____

_____

_____

_____

_____

_____

My world is resource rich. I find many ways to get the information and support I need. I live in total abundance.

See reference page regarding internet use

Anger Release

"For every minute you are angry you lose sixty seconds of happiness."

~Ralph Waldo Emerson

Many of us walk around, living our lives with an undercurrent of anger. This undercurrent does not discriminate, as we can be of any race, any educational level or wealth, of great fame, of any title, or own a successful business and still have this undercurrent running just below the surface. This anger could be formed from negative events in our lives, such as childhood abuse, abandonment, being overlooked for a promotion, responsibility for someone else's well-being, or from all of the chaos and injustice we hear daily in the media. Sometimes the observations of injustices gather slowly, swirling into a current of inner rage.

Most of us ignore this current, keeping it hidden and carefully contained, hoping it will go away. But it won't. It will eventually grow and show itself in the tone of our voices, the way we walk, the sharp flicker in our eyes, in our gestures, our facial expressions, and sometimes, in harsh words that slip out. In *The Artist's Way*, Julia Cameron writes, "Anger is our friend. Not a nice friend. Not a gentle friend. But a very, very loyal friend. It will always tell us when we have been betrayed. It will always tell us when we have betrayed ourselves. It will always tell us that it is time to act in our own best interest."

Anger is a gift if we listen and 1) honestly and objectively examine why we are angry by examining the experiences that helped to create this anger; 2) use tools, such as the exercises below, to release this anger; 3) discover what actions we need to take to live an authentic life filled with self-care and self-honor, in which this anger will dissipate; and 4) take action on these discoveries. Below are a few effective tools to use when we can feel anger beginning to surge within us:

Screaming into a Pillow

Scream into a soft pillow as loudly as possible; the pillow muzzles the sound, and no one will hear us.

Punching a Punching Bag

One of the best anger-release techniques wellness coaches use in therapy is punching bags. This is a great technique for caregivers, as well. Sometimes when we are in the midst of caregiving chaos, we may need a moment to release our anger safely. Excusing ourselves to punch a bag can feel very rewarding. We can just punch those bags until we are exhausted. Nobody gets physically or verbally hurt and we release the negative energy. There are different kinds of punching bags on the market. Discuss with specialists, which bags would work for you. The great tragedy with anger is not that we have it. The great tragedy is not listening to what it is trying to tell us and allowing it to build and stir. To become Inspired Caregivers, we must listen to our anger and release it.

Are you hiding or denying anger within your being? If so, are you willing to try these techniques to release it?

_____

_____

_____

_____

_____

_____

Expressing all emotions allows me to live more fully. I release my anger and frustration in healthy ways that free my spirit.

Insiders' Insights

Professionals Share Their Wisdom

"You, yourself, as much as anybody in the entire universe, deserve your love and affection."

~Buddha

We interviewed two very skilled and passionate professionals: Carol Metcalf, licensed marriage and family therapist, out of Santa Barbara, California, and Dr. Jill Tiongco, internal medicine physician, out of Carmel, California. They are instrumental to the health and well-being of both caregivers and their loved ones. It is our hope that the excerpts below bring awareness to the signs of overwhelm, and allow you to give yourself permission to sing, dance, love, laugh, and guiltlessly practice the art of self-care.

You Know You're in Overwhelm When:

Carol:

You're feeling exhausted and irritable, alternating with feelings of guilt attached to wanting a break from the caregiving role.

Dr. Jill Tiongco:

You're feeling irritable, anxious, you care too much or too little, see your own health decline, and feel indifferent.

If other people are saying, "How are you?" too often, chances are caregiver burnout is there.

What would you suggest caregivers do to take care of their physical, mental, and emotional health while caring for another?

Carol: Make time for self-care, take a walk, have lunch with a friend, and get support from friends, pastor, and family members. You need to claim proper nutrition and rest so you will not deplete yourself.

Dr. Jill Tiongco: Have your own personal physician. Make sure you have friends, friends, friends. Make sure you have your own "me time" from the beginning. If caregiver fatigue sets in, it might be too late.

If caregivers can only do one physical thing and one emotional thing to care for themselves while caring for another, what should it be?

Carol: Take time at different intervals in the day to relax, take a break, exercise, and get some fresh air. This helps the caregiver regroup physically and emotionally.

Dr. Jill Tiongco: Rest. Rest as much as possible. Do something that relieves your stress, be it yoga, exercising, or socializing.

One Last Word to Caregivers?

<u>Carol:</u> To be selfless and care for another is the most fulfilling thing a person can do in his or her lifetime.

<u>Dr. Jill Tiongco:</u> Caregivers, you are a gift to the world!

Their interviews can be read in their entireties at www.TheInspiredCaregiver.com.

What suggestions can you implement in your daily life?
In what ways can you reward yourself
for being "a gift to the world"?

_____

_____

_____

_____

My life is an example of how big love can be. When life sends me challenges, I see opportunities to grow, love, and be more than I ever imagined.

Mother Teresa of Calcutta: The Ultimate Inspired Caregiver

"It's not how much we give but how much love we put into the giving."

Mother Teresa

One day, when I was frustrated with Rose, feeling resentful of my many sacrifices, and bruised by her unkind words, I consulted my bookshelf to sip a sentence or two of encouragement. I asked God to lead me to a book that would ease my broken spirit. I closed my eyes and skimmed my fingers over my forgotten library of diverse books until one book felt good to me. When I opened my eyes, I was holding a book on Mother Teresa. As I started to browse through the pages, her words touched my soul and a deep peace oozed over my entire being. From that evening on, I returned again and again to her words, as it was my place of refuge. Not only did it give me the strength to care for Rose, it inspired me to do so from a place of patience and unconditional love.

Mother Teresa of Calcutta, India, could be considered one of the greatest Inspired Caregivers of all time. Although she didn't consider herself a caregiver, she cared for the dying, the leprous, the unwanted, the abandoned, and the unloved. She cleaned maggots from the bodies of the discarded and was sometimes not well received by the person in need. She witnessed horrendous human conditions that must have challenged the faith in which she walked.

By being an Inspired Caregiver, she understood the power of rest and rejuvenation on a daily basis. Although this book was not modeled after her life, her daily schedule consisted of many of the suggestions written in this book. According to the book *Loving Jesus*, edited by Jose' Luis Gonzalez-Balado and published by Franciscan Media (formerly St. Anthony Messenger Press), below is the daily schedule of Mother Teresa and her Sisters:

They begin each day with Mass, Holy Communion, and meditation. After Mass and breakfast, some of the Sisters go to the Home for Dying Destitutes, some to the leper colonies, and some to the little schools located in the slums. They go all over the city (in Calcutta alone, they have fifty-nine centers, the Home for Dying

Destitutes is only one center). They return around 12:30 p.m. and have lunch. After lunch, they do housework. Then, for half an hour, every Sister has to rest, because all the time they are on their feet. After, they have an examination of conscience, pray to the Liturgy of the Hours, and the Via Crucis, "Way of the Cross."

At 2 p.m., they have spiritual reading for half an hour, and then a cup of tea. At 3 p.m., the professed Sisters go out again. Between 6:15 p.m. and 6:30 p.m., everybody comes back home. From 6:30 p.m. to 7:30 p.m., they have adoration of the Blessed Sacrament. At 7:30 p.m., they have dinner. After dinner, for about twenty minutes, they have to prepare the work for the next morning. From 8:30 p.m. until 9 p.m., they have recreation. Everybody talks at the top of her lungs, after having worked all day long. At 9 p.m., they go to chapel for night prayers and prepare the meditations for the next morning.

Once a week, every week, they have a day of recollection. All the professed Sisters stay in for the day of recollection. This is the time they go to confession and spend more time in adoration of the Blessed Sacrament. It is a day they can regain their strength and fill their emptiness with Jesus. According to Mother Teresa, they can work ten to twelve hours a day in service to the poor, following this schedule.

Let us take a closer look at these Inspired Caregivers' daily lives:

- They meditate
- They Pray
- They have an effective, productive schedule.
- They fill their bodies up with the food it needs on a consistent basis.
- They exercise daily by mostly walking to their destinations.
- They take the time to rest.
- They feed their minds with empowering, spiritual material.
- They prepare and plan for the following day.
- They have recreational time in which they talk, laugh, and share with each other.
- They have a support system in each other.
- They release their pent-up energy and feelings in confession on a regular basis.
- They take one day out of the week to rejuvenate and regain their strength.

The Sisters have their own mantras that help them through the day and they remember why they do their work. As per Mother Teresa, no missionary of charity forgets the word of Christ: "I was hungry and you gave me food." When a Sister has a difficult time emotionally dealing with the great responsibility of this work, a Sister skilled in the area of counseling or the Mother Superior may counsel her.

Mother Teresa wrote letters to the late archbishop Ferdinand Perier of Calcutta and others. We could consider this journaling, as some of the letters revealed her darkest moments and feelings that she needed to express. Even Mother Teresa experienced dark emotions and feelings of unworthiness. We are not immune to this as well. It is important to have an outlet to release these feelings in a healthy manner to prevent destructive feelings of guilt and resentment, which can hold us captive.

When Mother Teresa was asked if she found it easy to carry out her work among the poor, she replied that it would not be easy without an intense life of prayer and a spirit of sacrifice. It should also be noted that Mother Teresa created a strong team to create and support the Missionaries of Charity.

Caregivers, although carrying a sometimes thankless, overwhelming, misunderstood responsibility, are doing honorable work that stands on a stage with those like Mother Teresa of Calcutta. No matter what religions we practice (if any), it is imperative that we follow effective, productive schedules and use the tools she used to give our loved ones the best care possible. By doing so, we create lives filled with inspiration and joy while we care for another.

Are you following the most efficient daily schedule that benefits both your health and the health of your loved one? If not, is there a technique Mother Teresa used that may be helpful to incorporate into your schedule?

_____

_____

_____

_____

_____

_____

My role as a caregiver is a sacred one! I follow an efficient schedule every day, which nourishes my mind, body, and soul.

Journaling

"Express yourself and allow time to be still."

"I can shake off everything as I write; my sorrows dis-appear, my courage is reborn."

~Anne Frank

Journaling, simply putting pen to paper, can be a healing experience. Devoting fifteen to twenty minutes each day to this practice can shift our outlook and give us the strength to be the supportive caregivers we desire to be. Journaling can be used to let go of thoughts and emotions that are bottled up inside. Treat yourself by using a special pen with which you love to write. Find a spot where you can be comfortable and alone. Light a candle, burn incense, or do anything that creates calm and allows you to focus. Sometimes the only refuge for freedom and privacy during journaling may be our cars.

You may find many emotions "stirred up" while journaling. Welcome and respect all that comes through this process. If you experience anger or frustration, acknowledge those feelings, and if you need to release them, hit a pillow or take a walk where no one can hear you and scream. Let your pen flow without censoring, releasing whatever wants to be released. It is not necessary to have something in mind that you want to write about, just start writing. Journaling can be an opportunity to celebrate your wins, document the hurdles you have overcome, and record the good things that happened in the course of your day. This can be a time to reconnect with your dreams and keep them alive. Your journal is for your eyes only, so be sure to find a safe place to store it. Don't filter what you write in fear that someone will read it. By using journaling as a part of your daily self-care practice, you can find the strength you need to spark your inspiration as you care for others.

Do you write in a journal daily? If not, is this something that you may enjoy?

_____

_____

_____

_____

_____

_____

Through every word I write, I allow a healthy release of my emotions. I allow time to quiet my mind in positive reflection.

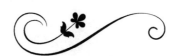

Develop the Art
of Gratitude

*"The more you praise and celebrate your life, the more
there is in life to celebrate."*

~Oprah Winfrey

While affirmations, prayers, and meditation are all
wonderful, highly effective tools for shifting our states
of mind, and therefore shifting our states of being, few
of us actually practice one of the most powerful shift-
ers of all: the art of gratitude. If we tread through our
days without awareness or reflection, thinking the same
frustrated thoughts and feeling the same negative feelings, we limit the experiences of the amazing lives we
are meant to have. Gratitude is one of the best tools
for connecting to just how rich our lives are. Consider

resting a moment to ponder all of the things for which we are grateful. Perhaps we are grateful for delicious cups of cappuccino, warm showers on cold mornings, satisfying meals, feeling good and having energy, being able to see the excited smiles on our grandchildren's faces, feeling the gentle touch of loved ones, walking through sweet, fragrant gardens, and hearing birds chanting sweet melodies outside our windows.

By conditioning our minds to focus on gratitude, we will notice how much our moods lift and how many more experiences that are gratifying come our way. All of the gifts we have been given will astonish us. Gratitude is like a muscle; the more we express it, the stronger and healthier we become. When we practice the art of gratitude upon awakening each morning, before eating each meal, and before laying our heads upon our pillows each evening, we may feel as if we have been reborn and replenished. Every day is a day to start over again—a brand new day.

In the midst of your caregiving journey, are you aware of the quiet blessings surrounding you? If not, will you accept our invitation to shift your everyday thoughts from what is wrong with your life to what is right with it? If so, start writing down five things for which you are grateful.

_____

_____

_____

_____

_____

_____

Everyday blessings surround me. I live in gratitude for all that is in my life.

Self-Care

"To keep a lamp burning we have to keep putting oil in it."

Mother Teresa

The Buddha taught that this is like this because that is like that. Because you smile, I am happy. This is like this; therefore, that is like that. And that is like that because this is like this. This is called dependent co-arising. My well-being, my happiness, depends very much on you and your well-being; your happiness depends upon me. I am responsible for you, and you are responsible for me. Anything I do wrong, you will suffer, and anything you do wrong, I have to suffer. Therefore, in order to take care of you, I have to take care of myself.

There is a story in the Pali Canon about a father and daughter who performed in the circus.

The father would place a very long bamboo stick on his forehead, and his daughter would climb to the top of the stick. When they did this, people gave them some money to buy rice and curry to eat. One day, the father told the daughter, "My dear daughter, we have to take care of each other. You have to take care of your father, and I have to take care of you, so that we will be safe. Our performance is very dangerous." Because if she fell, both would not be able to earn their living. If she fell, then broke her leg, they wouldn't have anything to eat. "My daughter, we have to take care of each other so we can continue to earn our living."

The daughter was wise. She said, "Father, you should say it this way: 'Each one of us has to take care of himself or herself, so that we can continue to earn our living.' Because during the performance, you take care of yourself, you take care of yourself only. You stay very stable, very alert. That will help me. And if when I climb I take care of myself, I climb very carefully, I do not let anything wrong happen to me. That is the way you should say it, Father, You take good care of yourself, and I take good care of myself. In that way we can continue to earn our living." The Buddha agreed that the daughter was right.

(Reprinted from Being Peace (1987) by Thich Nhat Hanh with permission of Parallax Press, Berkeley, California. www.parallax.org)

When we take care of ourselves with proper nutrition, rest, hydration, and exercise, we have more energy and patience. We feel better mentally, physically, and emotionally and are more productive and mindful of what we are doing in the moment. Everyone benefits when we are in balance. Like the father and daughter performers, it is extremely important for us to take care of ourselves so we can give our best to our love ones.

In what ways can you make self-care your priority?

_____

_____

_____

_____

I honor those I love and myself by taking care of me.
I make my health and well-being a priority.
All is well!

What Other Caregivers Do to Shake the Stress Off

We have spoken with thousands of caregivers and very few take care of themselves. When we come across Inspired Caregivers, we ask them what the secret to relieving their stress is. Below are a few of the answers we have received:

"I golf and beat the heck out of the golf ball, or I play with my grandchildren."

"I go to therapy weekly, and I'm attending Jin Shin Jyutsu, as well as meditation classes offered at my husband's medical center."

"I have pamper week. One day of the week I'll get a facial; the next week, I'll get a massage. It's my time."

"I walk my dog. I'm convinced that dogs are the best exercise machine there is!"

"My bible studies!"

"Dancing."

"Swimming in my pool."

"A weekly massage."

"Lunch with the girls."

"Yoga at my husband's medical facility."

"Bowling with the guys."

"I tend to my garden."

"My regular reading time!"

"My time is at the gym. I sweat out my frustrations."

"My family and friends are a great support. They listen and help me through it."

"Kick boxing."

"My on-line, caregiving support group."

What brings you joy? Do you have an outlet to release your stress? If not, what activities will make your heart

sing? When will you give yourself permission to participate in these activities?

_____

_____

_____

_____

_____

_____

I have released any burdens, and I feel light and free. Stress has left my body; I am calm, and all is as it should be.

The Inspired Caregiver Checklist

YES	NO	The Inspired Caregiver Checklist:
❑	❑	Do you have a strong foundation and an organized system that can be duplicated?
❑	❑	Did you create your Inspired Caregiver Team, and are you utilizing their talents consistently?
❑	❑	Do you have a team of supportive friends and family members?
❑	❑	Do you have at least one individual on your team who can care for your loved one without your supervision when needed?

YES   NO

❑   ❑   Do you exercise at least three times a week for twenty minutes on a consistent basis?

❑   ❑   Do you eat healthy, nutritious foods consistently (*preferably organic*)?

❑   ❑   Do you receive the right amount of rest for your body consistently every evening?

❑   ❑   Do you drink 64 ounces of filtered water daily *(or the daily requirement needed for your body)*?

❑   ❑   Do you take time off weekly for your personal care?

❑   ❑   Do you have boundaries? Do you honor them consistently?

❑   ❑   Do you have many healthy avenues to release your daily stress?

❑   ❑   Do you laugh often?

❑   ❑   Are you listening to and/or reading empowering, humorous, and/or healing material on a regular basis?

YES   NO

❏   ❏   Are you journaling your thoughts and feelings on a consistent basis?

❏   ❏   Do you experience moments of joy in your everyday life?

❏   ❏   Did you create a sacred space where you can pray, breathe, meditate, visualize, or just "be" on a daily basis?

❏   ❏   Do you have a safe, private space where you can release your negative, frustrated, pent-up energy by punching a punching bag, screaming into a pillow, or participating in a vigorous exercise, such as boxing or kickboxing?

If you have answered yes to the questions above, you will have greater endurance, patience, compassion, and joy for every single day given to you. You will live an inspired, rich life filled with endless possibilities and new awakenings. You will have become an Inspired Caregiver!

Sweet Surrender...Create Your Exit Plan

"The number one reason a person will be taken out of a home care situation and placed into a facility is due to caregiver burnout."

~Christopher & Dana Reeve Foundation

What do we do if we have done everything on the Inspired Caregiver Checklist consistently and are still in overwhelm? Then it is time to sit down, inhale a big, beautiful breath of life-giving oxygen, hold it ever so gently, and slowly release it, along with all of our burdens, worries, unrealistic expectations, pride, and fear. It is time to surrender. Our work here is done.

Along with surrendering our responsibilities, we must surrender caring about what our loved ones, friends, and family members think about our decision, especially if they have not been in the caregiving trenches with us. They cannot possibly understand the emotional, physical, and mental pressure we have had to endure. Terry Cole-Whittaker's book *What You Think of Me is None of My Business* appropriately states what we can proudly proclaim. It is a good idea to adopt this statement as our personal mantra while going through the process of surrendering.

We must also surrender our pride and belief that we are the only people who can care for our loved ones properly. What we refuse to recognize emotionally within ourselves will manifest in our bodies eventually, leaving us no choice but to surrender. We can create an exit plan with our Inspired Caregiver Teams. There may be many options available, such as placing our loved ones in facilities that specialize in their individual needs, or allowing a qualified sibling to take over indefinitely.

If our decision to surrender throws us into emotional chaos, remember this quote by Chinese philosopher Lao Tzu: "Muddy water. Let stand. Becomes clear." If we give ourselves time to think through our decisions, we will see that someone other than us can care for our loved ones efficiently. Those who disagree with our decisions, including our loved ones, most likely will eventually understand, and our worlds will become clear once more. Day by day, we will awaken to inspiration again and eventually discover that the life we saved was our own.

Our reluctance to surrender while in overwhelm can endanger our loved one's health, erasing all of the progress we may have made. *Are you willing to surrender your caregiving responsibilities to someone else? When and with whom will you start creating your exit plan?*

I surrender any guilt or shame. I know there is honor in releasing to the universe that which is no longer mine. By my surrendering, I am giving a gift to those in my care and to myself.

Assisted Living

When the needs are more than you can provide

"The best thing we can give the public is education about planning when we can no longer care for ourselves. Who will care for us and what assisted living facility should we go to when our care becomes too great?"

Nerissa Ramos

On our caregiving journeys, we may agonize over the question of whether or not to place our loved ones in assisted living facilities when the care needed has become too great. Nerissa Ramos, BSN, registered nurse, and co-owner of Anjelica's Villa Assisted Residential Care in Seaside, California, is passionate about her field. She sheds light on this sometimes-feared subject.

According to Nerissa, the best time to place our loved ones in assisted living facilities is when our loved ones need supervision 24-7. Signs additional care is needed are:

- When they no longer care about their grooming

- When they have a hard time taking their medications at certain times and/or taking the correct dose

- When they stop eating

- When they dress inappropriately or consistently wear dirty clothes

- When they become difficult

"Let us face the issue," Nerissa states matter-of-factly. "No matter how mentally alert we are, sometimes physically we can't do it. It's part of life: we need to eat, we need to bathe, and we need to do all these things."

If our loved ones do not want to be placed in assisted living facilities, we need to think of the safety of our loved ones. Our consciences may haunt us if we do not put their safety first and something really bad happens. Nerissa suggests that we work with their medical doctors for guidance.

Much of the time, our families complicate the matter by being in denial and making excuses for our loved ones. According to Nerissa, a change in our loved ones' daily routines is the most crucial time. "So many times we ignore it. For example, a husband responds to his wife sleeping in until noon when she has never done that before, "Oh, well, she's just tired. She needs her sleep. She needs a break." This happens until it becomes a pattern, and she declines. We do not help our loved ones by being in denial and making excuses. By doing this, we hurt our loved ones, and put others in danger as well."

When we asked Nerissa if we should feel guilty, Nerissa responded that guilt is inevitable, but she believed that early education is most important. If we are educated, we will not want to burden our families with our illnesses if we have become too much for them to care for.

"I know they will feel guilty somehow. But, like my children, they have their own lives. If my children put me in a home, I don't want them to feel guilty. I will say to them that I guess this is the time. If this is the time, this is the time. I'm going to tell them not to feel guilty about it. This is a part of life that we should not feel guilty about. We want our loved ones to have the best care possible when it has become too much in our lives. It is a part of the cycle of life. This is why it is important to have our wishes known to our children. We need open communication to whomever we think will be looking after us when we grow old. Having a living will, advanced directive is very important. Public education is the most important thing. Education is needed. When it is time, it is time. Preparing for this day is important."

Nerissa's interview can be read in its entirety at www.TheInspiredCaregiver.com.

*Have you thought about what should be done if you can
no longer care for yourself? Have you communicated
your wishes with your loved ones, should the burden of
caring for you become too great? If your loved one's
care is too great, have you thought about the possibility
of placing him or her in an assisted living facility? Why
and why not? Write down the thoughts that come to
your mind when presented with these questions:*

---

*I am releasing any thoughts of guilt or shame.
I am making decisions that best serve my loved ones
and my well-being.*

Caregiver Affirmations

We Celebrate You!
Read this aloud at least once every
morning with feeling!

(You are programming your subconscious mind to become an Inspired Caregiver.)

Today is the first day of the rest of my life, and every minute is a chance to start over again.

I focus only on the positive and on the solutions.

I am a kind, loving, and patient person.

I am an excellent caregiver, and what I do is needed and wanted.

Those in my care get the most gentle and loving care!

I know the healthier I am physically, emotionally, spiritually, and mentally, the easier it is to care for my loved one and the healthier they become.

I eat healthy, well-balanced meals daily, and I get plenty of rest every night.

I always fill myself with good motivational and spiritual material to keep me strong and inspired!

It is important for me to take care of myself while caring for another.

I am a beautiful person inside and out.

What other people think of me is none of my business. What is important is what I think of myself, and I am good.

I take consistent time out for rejuvenating and relaxing activities.

I look to each day with excitement and enthusiasm; every day is a good day!

To watch the video affirmations, please visit:
TheInspiredCaregiver.com

Serenity Prayer

God grant me the serenity

to accept the things I cannot change,

Courage to change the things I can,

and the wisdom to know the difference.

Resources

The resources below are discussed in this book. For a list of caregiving organizations and support groups, please visit www.TheInspiredCaregiver.com.

Inspired wellness coaches available for caregiving counsel via telephone and sessions are:

Carol A. Metcalf, LMFT   Santa   Barbara,   CA
805-280-5389

Donna Wood, M.A., LMFT Santa Cruz and SF Bay Area, CA 831-566-2696 www.DonnaWoodmft.com

www.TheInspiredCaregiver.com Download your free Medical Alert Card template

www.TheInspiredCeo.com - Consulting and coaching. For assistance with creating a life of bliss regardless of your circumstance http://www.dol.gov/whd/fmla/ Look into the Family and Medical Leave Act (FMLA)

www.ChristopherReeve.org Christopher and Dana Reeve Foundation

http://www.TonyRobbins.com/ Peak Performance strategist and author, Anthony Robbins

www.CherylRichardson.com Author of the book *The Art of Extreme Self-Care*

www.SteveChandler.com Author of the book *Time Warrior*

www.AnjelicasVilla.com Owned by the Ramos Family (Assisted Residential Care)

www.Presto.com Use email with loved ones who do not use a computer or the internet

www.TheInspiredCaregiver.com
Watch Inspired Caregiver affirmation video

www.Youtube.com Watch instructional, comedy, and inspirational videos, and find helpful resources

Inspired Books to Read:

The Everything Green Smoothies Book, by Britt Brandon, with Lorena Novak Bull, RD
Time Warrior, by Steve Chandler
Sabbath, by Wayne Muller
Being Peace, by Thich Nhat Hanh, edited by Arnold Kotler
The Artist Way, by Julia Cameron
The Sound of Paper, by Julia Cameron
Dying To Be Me, by Anita Moorjani
What You Think of Me Is None of My Business, by Terry Cole-Whittaker

(Please visit www.TheInspiredCaregiver.com for a list of empowering books.)

Recommendations that May Work for You:

The Next Best Thing to Fruits & Vegetables

It can be difficult to consume the amount of fruits and vegetables your body needs.

Good nutrition takes time and planning. Clinically proven Juice Plus+® helps you bridge the gap between the 7 to 13 servings of fruits and vegetables recommended by The United States Department of Agriculture (USDA) and the nutrition you actually get with your busy schedule. www.caregiverfueljuiceplus.com

To grow your own organic fruits and vegetables, consider Tower Garden. Find out more at: https://caregiverfuel.towergarden.com/

References

Please read before setting up your banking on-line, purchasing on Amazon.com, or setting up your Facebook account:

We strongly suggest you consult a certified security computer specialist to protect your computer from hackers, viruses, spyware, and other malicious software. At the time of this printing, the Geek Squad, affiliated with Best Buy, has certified security computer specialists who can help set up your computer systems. Avoid banking or doing anything that requires you to use your name and password at public internet hotspots (available at coffee shops, libraries, hotels, bookstores, etc.) for the same reasons.

*Please, be mindful of what you write on Facebook.

Wellness Coaches and Confidentiality

There are some exceptions to confidentiality. Wellness coaches (mental health professionals) are required by law to report reasonable suspicions of child abuse, adult physical abuse, or suspicion of hurting yourself or someone else unless protective measures are taken. If confidentiality is of great concern, you can always go to the Board of Psychology in your state to discover the laws that govern confidentiality with your wellness coach. Also, it is a good idea to read any release form before signing it, as it may give permission to release private information to a third party, such as your insurance companies.

"Are You a Caregiver," Definition of Caregiver from the 1993 Random House Webster's Dictionary, Executive Director: Sol Steinmetz, Project Editor: Carol G. Braham, published by Ballantine Books, a division of Random House, Inc.

"I Didn't Sign Up for This," *Time Warrior*, by Steve Chandler, published by Maurice Bassett

"Boundaries," Definition of boundary from the 1993 Random House Webster's Dictionary, Executive Director: Sol Steinmetz, Project Editor: Carol G. Braham, published by Ballantine Books, a division of Random House, Inc.

"Therapy – The New Black," *Dying to Be Me*, by Anita Moorjani, published by Hayhouse Publishing

"Breathe," Anthony Robbins personal achievement system "Personal Power," © *Robbins Research International, Inc.*

"Nutrition! No Ifs, Ands, or Buts. It's a Must," *Everything Green Smoothies Book*, by Britt Brandon, with Lorena Novak Bull, RD, published by Adams Media, a division of F+W Media, Inc.

"Give Yourself Permission to Cry," *The Sound of Paper*, by Julia Cameron, published by Jeremy P. Tarcher/Penguin, a member of the Penguin Group (USA) Inc.

"Anger Release," *The Artist Way*, by Julia Cameron, published by Jeremy P. Tarcher/Penguin, a member of the Penguin Group (USA) Inc.

"Mother Teresa of Calcutta: The Ultimate Caregiver," *Loving Jesus*, edited by Jose' Luis Gonzalez-Balado, published by Franciscan Media (formerly St. Anthony Messenger Press)

"Self-Care," *Being Peace* (1987), by Thich Nhat Hanh, with permission of Parallax Press, Berkeley, California, www.parallax.org

Acknowledgements

Peggi would like to thank:

God, Jesus, and the whole God team.

Sheila Shaw (Carter), for your rock-solid support and your brilliant mind and talent. I am forever grateful to you for helping me set up the foundation for Rose and for carrying much of my burden. I know it wasn't easy.

Tia Walker, for believing in me, for your commitment, and for being a beautiful example of a truly inspired individual! If Pollyanna had a sister, she would be you!

Jeannie Shaw (Jene'), for never-ending positive support and love!

Eve, for always being with me.

Louis Gonzales, for unconditional love and always making me laugh. I miss you so much!

Dr. Jill Tiongco, for invaluable guidance and for being an Inspired Physician!

Lisa and Gonzalo Jaquez, for being incredible examples of Inspired Caregivers and for being the change you would like to see in this world! You two are so inspirational.

Donna Wood, for sincere support and guidance, and for being a brilliant example of an Inspired Caregiver and "wellness coach!"

Sharon Law Tucker, for being you: authentic, supportive, caring, and inspiring!

Ruth-de-toot-toot, for sharing your love of life with me.

Kathleen Ross, Anne Ashley, and Libby Stanton for giving us honest, powerful feedback, and of course, for your unconditional love and support! IAOOTLSITU

Brenna Stanton for your enthusiasm, excellent feedback, and loving support! We love your ideas, and I am amazed by your natural writing ability! I love your writing and your heart!

Nerissa, Benjamin, and all the wonderful caregivers at Anjelica's Villa: You are all my angels, especially you, Nerissa! What a gift you have been to me!

Tran Salim, for your friendship, ear, wisdom, and great sense of humor!

Mary Margareht Rose, for your great love and light.

Carol Metcalf and Maryjean Ballner, for your wonderful contributions to this book.

Ruth Wishengrad and Hugh Browne, for your support and sharing your gifts of photography with us!

Sandra Haven at SC Studios, for your sincere support and gifts of love and beauty.

Hope Tadema, for your support and great humor.

Cathy Espitia, for your prayers, beautiful cards, and loving support.

Meryn Gruhn Di Tullio for your kind support, great depth, and great humor.

Kita, for your love and inspiration.

My huge, supportive family and friends including Ethel, Claude, Brandon, Lindsey, Danielle, Brian, Devon, Jeremy, Taylor, Leah, Kristine, Aaron, Jay, Bill, Kathy, Mark, and Janice for your love, support, great meals, inspiration, and laughter! "My cup runneth over!"

To the thousands of caregivers who have shared your hearts with me throughout the years: Don't ever forget "You are a gift to the world!"

To all of the beautiful individuals I mentioned above and to those of you I missed:

Somewhere in my youth or childhood, I must have done something good to have had your help carrying me through this intense journey of caregiving. I would especially like to thank Rose who, if she had not granted me the honor of caring for her, I would have never had the whispered rewards and profound awakenings I experienced on the emotional rollercoaster of caring for a loved one suffering from dementia.

Tia's heartfelt appreciation goes out to:

My mother Emma and my father Roger; I am eternally grateful to you for being my biggest cheering committee throughout my life and for being ordinary people with extraordinary hearts.

The best sons in the world: Ashleigh, Nolan, and Brenton, who inspired me daily and are the wind beneath my wings.

Gregory Jones, for being a dear heart brother and positive, supportive force even when life threw curve balls.

Peggi Speers, for being an angel, sister, friend, and inspirational pillar in my life.

Sheila Shaw, a kindred soul sister who encouraged and believed in the book and me.

My family, whose love transcends space and time.

Jeni Ambrose and Diana Estrada, who have been close witnesses, held space for me, and shared wisdom.

Maryjean Ballner, for your editing finesse and giving heart.

Carol Metcalf, for your compassion, beauty, and sense of humor.

Matthew Patton for your vision, support, account-ability, and love.

Hugh Browne, for your awesome photography and joyful spirit.

Ruth Wishengrad, for your kind heart, photography, and ability to capture a magical moment.

To the many caregivers who shared their lives and stories and do the often thankless job of caring for another.

I have been graced with beautiful friends, family members, and community. Your love, support, and encouragement helped me to be strong during my time of loss. Thank you to those whose names may not appear here, but who have been a part of my journey. I hold you in my heart in deep appreciation.

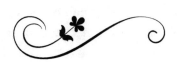

About the Author

Peggi Speers

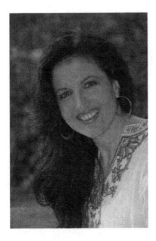

Peggi Speers has a passionate desire to convey the truths and techniques she learned during her journey as a caregiver. While caring for loved ones with cancer, kidney failure, stroke, and dementia, she experienced both the benefits of self-care and the trials of self-neglect.

As cofounder of Patient's Pride, Inc., a company that specializes in custom catheter support systems, which protect the health and comfort of clients with peritoneal dialysis catheters, insulin pumps, and feeding tubes, Peggi has always reached beyond phone lines and emails to encourage clients contending with medical needs, as well as those devoted to caring for them. After speaking with thousands of caregivers throughout the United States and Canada, she decided to co-create a comforting, empowering book that she wished had been available during her own journey.

Music is another outlet of creative expression. Peggi Speers has co-written numerous songs featured on television programs such as *MTV—Making the Band*, *Women of Desperate Housewives*, *Sex and the City*, *Chicken Soup for the Soul,* Fox *Sports*, *The Maury Povich Show*, *The Young and the Restless*, *Access Hollywood*, *Guiding Light*, Comcast *Sports*, *Another World*, and many others.

About the Author

Tia Walker

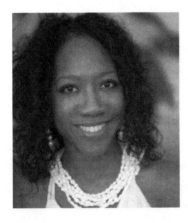

Armed with more than two decades of business management and marketing experience, **Tia Walker** founded The Inspired CEO, an executive coaching and consulting firm. Tia believes that we are each the CEOs of our lives and are empowered to make the work that we do serve as an inspiration to others. A believer in the vastness of the human spirit, Tia has developed coaching programs that combine personal development, work satisfaction, and an element of service. Her often sold-out retreats encourage participants to get out of their routines and experience personal rejuvenation and business transformation.

She is a highly sought after emcee, hosting numerous events including Silicon Valley Women's Initiative Entrepreneur of the Year Awards at Google, to Community Action Commission's Distinguished "Champions" Awards of Santa Barbara County. Tia is an experienced speaker, delivering messages to audiences from 5-5000.

Tia takes the same approach to being an Inspired Caregiver. She believes that whatever you do, you can do it in joy and with love.

As an entrepreneur who built her own successful consulting business, she also empathetically helps other business owners and professionals set priorities and create the balance they want between life and work. She lights up while assisting organizations and individuals interested in becoming catalysts of change. One of her most provocative messages is about living a congruent life, both personally and professionally. Tia has assisted her clients in creating "blissful lives."

Tia enjoys reading, dancing, hooping, gardening, traveling, and people in general. She is the proud mother of three sons: Ashleigh, Nolan, and Brenton.

Caregiver Stress Relief

Even with our best efforts, sometimes our role as caregiver gets the best of us and we are overwhelmed and stressed.

We would like to offer you a **FREE REPORT**
7 Steps for Caregiver Stress Relief

If you are interested in receiving a copy, we will be happy to e-mail it to you. Send an email to: FreeReport@TheInspiredCaregiver.com with
CAREGIVER RELIEF in the subject line.

Made in the USA
Lexington, KY
28 January 2018